FROM RELUCTANT
RUNNER TO GUINNESS
WORLD RECORD BREAKER

BEYOND IMPOSSIBLE

MIMI ANDERSON

WITH LUCY WATERLOW

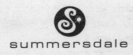

summersdale

CONTENTS

PROLOGUE

I had never been in so much pain – and for me, that's saying something. After all, I have run for 156 miles through the Sahara desert in 50°C heat when dehydrated and weak. I have run alone non-stop pulling a sledge for six days over ice in the Arctic, facing a wind chill of –70°C. I have given birth three times. But the pain of all those experiences is nothing compared to how I felt now running – or more like limping – towards Land's End in Cornwall in the darkness and pouring rain.

Everything hurt from my bruised and swollen arm to my sore, blistered feet. After years of competing in ultra-distance races, I have become accustomed to the onset of pain and adept at pushing myself to continue when my body is screaming that it has had enough. This time felt different, perhaps I had finally found my limit.

I must have looked like something from *The Walking Dead* as I dragged my battered body along the road, occasionally moaning in pain. The only way to alleviate the excruciating agony I felt burning in every limb was to stop running. But stopping wasn't an option. I was on the cusp of achieving my dream of gaining a Guinness World Record, and I couldn't give up now.

Twelve days earlier I had set off on fresh legs from John o'Groats in Scotland full of enthusiasm and energy. I was aiming to become the fastest female to run the length of Great Britain. But nearly 840 miles later, I was sleep-deprived, drained and exhausted. I needed to maintain a certain pace to achieve the record but moving at all was becoming increasingly difficult.

There was only one mile to go to reach the finish line but it felt like one hundred. I had run through Britain's hottest summer for decades, been struck by a car and held up by an overzealous police officer to reach this point. Even though I was now so close to my goal, I didn't feel I could take another step.

My husband, Tim, was cycling beside me shouting words of encouragement and trying to distract me from the pain.

'Come on, Mimi, keep going, you're nearly there, you can do it,' he said.

I should have felt grateful for his encouragement but instead I felt grumpy and resentful.

Easy for you to say sitting there on your bum on your bike, I thought. *You try running with legs like lead, burning feet and an injured arm.*

My body was finding various ways to tell me that it couldn't go on. I had a headache, my vision was blurry, my stomach was sore and, thanks to the weather, I was soaked to the bone. All my muscles hurt but in particular the ligaments and tendons in my left foot were screaming for attention, as they were badly damaged and weak. Every time I took a step and landed on the tarmac road, the impact sent shooting pains up my leg and I felt as though my ankle was going to give way beneath me. I kept hobbling along and tried to find any reason I could to stop, even if only for a few precious seconds – to alleviate the agony I was in. I paused to fiddle with my trainer laces, to scratch my leg or to readjust my clothing, any excuse for a break.

By now, Tim was becoming increasingly frustrated with me. I was going so slowly, he had to dismount his bike and walk beside me. Then to his dismay, I stopped again – and this time I had no intention of continuing. I simply couldn't take another step.

'I can't do it,' I told Tim as I swayed by the roadside on my wobbly legs. 'I can't go any further. It hurts too much.'

'Don't be ridiculous!' he replied, aghast at my decision. 'You can't give up now! Do you realise you are only a mile from the finish? You have run for 839 miles, you just need to keep moving and manage another one!'

I know it wasn't rational to have come this far only to throw the towel in with a mile to go, but by this point I wasn't thinking straight; I was too tired and in so much pain. For the previous 12 mornings, I had risen at 4.30 a.m. after four hours' sleep, pulled on my trainers and started running. I had run two and a half back-to-back marathons a day for nearly a fortnight. I was now completely and utterly spent and all I wanted to do was stop.

At that moment I no longer cared about gaining a world record. I didn't consider how much I had sacrificed and how much I had given to reach this point. My mind was in survival mode and was only certain about one thing – I had to stop running.

'Tell the rest of the crew it's over; they need to come and get me,' I told Tim, referring to the rest of my team who had trailed me in two motorhomes throughout my journey. They had gone ahead to the finish line where they were waiting for me along with other supporters, local press and the mayor of Land's End. They had all gathered to cheer me on for the final 100 metres and were ready and waiting for the guest of honour, holding up tape made from pink toilet paper for me to break as I crossed the finish line. But I wasn't going to make it to the party.

As I stood catching my breath and feeling some relief from standing still instead of running, I looked at Tim and saw he looked as sleep-deprived as I felt. He had dark, puffy bags under his bloodshot eyes and looked drawn and exhausted. He had taken time off work to support my run and instead of having a relaxing break away from his job, he had been snatching a few hours' sleep in a motorhome, cycling beside me for miles and ensuring my needs for food and water were met – often without much gratitude. I had mostly only been able to grunt thanks as food and water was handed to me as I ran, or complained when I was told I had to run faster to stay on target. He had done it and put up with my mood because he knew how much it meant to me to complete this challenge and achieve a world record.

'You've come so far, Mimi,' he told me. 'One more mile and you could be a world-record holder! One more mile and then you can stop and celebrate and all this will have been worth it.'

Then he added: 'Don't think you can give up now and try again next year as we can't go through all this again!'

This was actually spoken with a number of expletives I won't add here but you get the idea, he wasn't going to let me quit with such a short distance to go. While I hate to admit my husband is ever right, in this instance, he was right. This was my second attempt at achieving a world record and I might never make it this far again. I knew too well that just making it to the start line was a challenge in itself and even with the best-laid plans, things can, and will, go wrong along the way.

After all the preparation and the pain, I had made it to Cornwall and I couldn't quit now. I wouldn't just be letting myself down but Tim and the rest of my crew who had worked tirelessly to get me to this point. They had believed in me and supported me, stepping away from their own lives for a fortnight to help me achieve this crazy goal I had set myself. It wasn't as if I was an Olympian with the hopes of a nation riding on my success. This challenge had been for me and me alone, and the crew had done what they could to help, with nothing to gain for themselves. They had given their time and support for me. So now I had to finish for them.

I resumed my painful plod, dragging one foot in front of the other as Tim got back on his bike beside me.

Just one more mile. One more mile. I can do this, I thought over and over trying to keep my body in a rhythm and block out the pain.

As my mind got back to the task in hand, I realised the self-imposed delay had cost me minutes I couldn't afford to lose. There was only a mile to go but time was precious, and more importantly, running out. I was going slower than a sloth – would I be able to make it to the finish in time to break the world record?

CHAPTER ONE

FROM RELUCTANT RUNNER TO ULTRA-FIT

Day one: John o'Groats to Tain, 85 miles

The journey had begun 840 miles north of Land's End, 12 days earlier. My friend Becky Healey had nudged me awake at 5 a.m., rousing me from a restless night's sleep. We had spent the night in a motorhome, which would be our home for nearly a fortnight. As I lay in bed, I could hear strong winds blowing around outside the van in its exposed position on the tip of Great Britain. The seemingly gale-force gusts had rattled the sides of the vehicle all night. But even if conditions had been perfect, I doubt I would have slept better. I had been tossing and turning worrying about the challenge I was about to face.

It would have been all too easy to roll over and go back to sleep, but then I remembered where I was and what lay ahead. It was days before my 46th birthday, and while other people may have jetted away on holiday to celebrate the occasion or thrown a party, I was going to attempt to run into the record books. From my starting point in John o'Groats, I planned to run 840 miles to Land's End, faster than a woman had ever run it before.

Becky and the other members of my crew would be responsible for my timekeeping and she wasn't going to let me get behind on day one.

'Come on, Mimi, time to get up,' she said, giving me a prod. Although I didn't appreciate being awoken at that moment, Becky's strict punctuality was exactly what was needed and why I had wanted her to be on board. We had met through running and, as a natural leader, who runs her own accountancy business, she was the perfect person to keep my challenge on track. Becky is always mega-efficient and super-organised so I was delighted when she had offered to join my crew after she heard I was attempting a world record. Knowing someone so diligent was managing my timekeeping was one less thing for me to worry about. She also knew exactly what to say to keep me motivated. Even though I had been training for months to prepare for what lay ahead of me, being told you have to get up and run 840 miles is a daunting prospect. If Becky had said: 'Time to get up and go for an 840-mile run,' I would certainly have stayed in bed. Having crewed on ultra-races before (an ultra is deemed anything over the marathon distance of 26.2 miles), she knew the right words to use and what I needed to hear. To face this arduous journey, I would have to break it up into stages and just focus on making it to the end of each day.

'Tain, here we come,' she said. The scenic, historic town in the Highlands would be our first overnight stop – a mere 85 miles away.

Just why had I decided to try to become the fastest woman in the world to run the length of Britain? Well, whenever I am asked 'why?' my usual response is 'why not?' And this is exactly what I thought about tackling JOGLE as it is known (or the Gallic sounding LE JOG, if you go south to north), when a friend had suggested it to me after I had completed a number of other ultra-races. I thought about it and I couldn't think of a single reason why not. I'm a strong believer that you need to challenge yourself in life and shouldn't be afraid to take on something that scares you. Failure isn't something I am afraid of. How can we ever know what it is possible to achieve unless we try?

The history of the event also appealed to me. People had been trying to set records for travelling the length of Britain in weird and wonderful ways since the 1800s. Some had cycled it, some had travelled on unicycles, one even did it in a motorised bathtub. But I, like a brave (and perhaps a little crazy) few before me, wanted to run it.

The route would involve travelling from John o'Groats down through Scotland to the Lake District, then passing through Preston, Shrewsbury and into Wales via Chepstow.

I'd then cross over the Severn Bridge back into England to run through Somerset and Devon, eventually entering Cornwall and running all the way down to Land's End. The previous record set in 2006 stood at 12 days, 16 hours and 23 minutes. In order to beat it, I would have to stick to a strict schedule of running at a decent pace, with minimal time 'wasted' to rest and recover. My crew and I decided to break the days up into four four-hour stints of running with no more than an hour break in between, when I could rest, eat or get a massage. This meant after the first day, I would be awoken at 4.30 a.m. so I could get going at 5 a.m., running in the four-hour blocks till I could stop to sleep around midnight. My crew would have to be very bossy about getting me to keep to the schedule as much as possible, as every minute counted towards getting the record.

On the first day, I had been afforded a lie-in as my world-record attempt would start at 7.15 a.m. Thanks to Becky's wake-up call, I was on schedule. She handed me a coffee and a smoothie to drink and then, like a knight going into battle, I pulled on my athletic armour – three-quarter-length leggings, a long-sleeve running top and a high-vis waistcoat over the top for safety, not forgetting to pin my 'lucky charm' to my sports bra, a brooch my godmother had given me when I was christened, which I wear in all my races. I pulled my blonde hair out of my face with a headband in my favourite colour of pink and laced up my trainers. I was ready to go.

Opening the motorhome door I was greeted by a crisp July morning. The sun was just beginning to peep over the horizon and it promised to be a fine summer's day.

'Morning, Mimi,' said my friend Phil Bullen, the second member of my crew, as he emerged from our neighbouring motorhome. 'Are you ready to run?'

Phil is a police officer and keen ultrarunner who had also offered to join my crew after hearing about my world-record attempt. He was an asset to the team, as well as being lovely company – I knew his strong, authoritative presence would make me feel safer when he accompanied me on sections of the route I might otherwise have felt apprehensive about running through alone, especially in the evenings when it would be dark. He was also an excellent map reader, which was essential, as I couldn't afford to waste time getting lost and going off track if I wanted to gain the record.

As well as Becky and Phil, my good friend Karyn Moore, who I have known since I was 23 years old when we met through our husbands, was also part of the crew. She is a warm, smiley person who loves to talk and get to know people. She chats constantly, asking so many questions, finding out everything there is to know about someone within half an hour of meeting them. I knew her endless entertaining chatter would be a distraction to take my mind off the pain as the challenge went on.

My fourth crew member, Alan Young, was an old hand at JOGLE as he had been part of the crew when the existing record had been set by Sharon Gayter in 2006. As she had set the mark with his help, he knew exactly what I would have to do to beat it. He took his role very seriously and I knew his professionalism and experience would bolster my record attempt further.

Finally, my husband, Tim, would be joining us on day eight. I wasn't entirely happy about this initially as he had never been involved in my racing before and had never crewed. Although he was well-qualified having served in the Army with the Queen's Own Highlanders for five years, I was concerned his emotional attachment as my husband would prevent him being an effective member of the crew, and he could end up being more of a hindrance than a help. Would he be able to push me to keep going when the going got tough and he saw how much pain I was in? After a number of arguments, we reached a compromise and decided he would join me – but only for the final five days, enabling me to get into a routine and push my worries about how he would cope to the back of my mind at the start of the run.

Having a well-organised, supportive crew is crucial to success in many ultra-distance events, and especially when attempting to run a world record. The crew would follow me on the whole journey in the two motorhomes we'd hired, taking it in turns to cycle behind me or run beside me (as per the Guinness rules, they were never allowed to cycle in front of me), ensuring I was happy, fed and watered. A vital part of their job was keeping a logbook of the journey, noting every time I stopped for a break and when I started up again. The distances I covered in each section and the length of time taken for each break all had to be recorded. At every opportunity, they had to obtain witness statements from the general public, asking them to sign forms confirming they had seen me run past them, giving their name, location and the time they had seen me. This would all be used as evidence to ratify a new world record – should I be lucky enough to achieve that goal. Guinness World Records criteria are very strict, so no stone could be left unturned in gathering evidence of my epic run.

As well as being unable to prove a record without my crew, I quite simply wouldn't be able to do it without them. They would be my rocks, allowing me to focus on running while they sorted everything else – meals, massages, map reading, laundry, emptying the motorhome loos, refuelling. Their work was relentless. On top of all that, they would provide the support, encouragement and, at times, light relief I would need to keep me going. Such is the organisation and constant support needed, Becky has often told me crewing an ultra can be harder than actually running one!

With my crew assembled for JOGLE, I then had to plot my route and overnight stops. I decided to start in Scotland instead of Cornwall for a number of reasons. Firstly, somehow it seemed psychologically easier to run 'down' south rather than 'up' north. The previous record had been set doing it the other way round, and I was concerned that if I followed the same pattern, I would constantly be comparing my times to where Sharon had been at each stage, which could prove to be demoralising and distracting – it would be far better just to focus on what I was doing. Thirdly, as I am a Scot, I wanted to start the run in Scotland so I would be running through my home turf, where friends and family in the area would be able to come to cheer me on, when I felt fresh. I knew the longer the challenge went on, the more tired and grumpy I would get, so I would rather see friends and family when I still had the energy to fully show my gratitude for their support.

The final reason for doing it this way round was to banish the memory of a failed attempt to break the record the year before. I had tried to do it in 2007 starting at Land's End and running north but I was forced to pull out in the early stages due to injury. Towards the end of the first day, I'd felt as though my knee was going to give way but I chose to ignore it. By the second day, it had become so bad I was struggling to run at all and had to resort to walking. Setting out on the third day, I then began to develop a niggling pain in my hip joint as well, so that even walking became painful. I knew it didn't feel right and that I couldn't ignore these issues any longer. I went to see a physiotherapist, who confirmed my worst fears. She told me there was a serious issue with my pyriformis, a muscle situated in my bottom, and if I continued running on it for another nine days, I could make it even worse and risk further injury, possibly preventing me from ever being able to run long distances again.

I wasn't ready to admit defeat yet so after her treatment, she asked me to try a run outside her building. I barely managed a step, as my hip was so sore. I was devastated, I felt as though I was a complete fraud – who did I think I was trying to run the length of the country? I couldn't even manage to jog across a car park. It took ten minutes until I eventually conceded – it was over. With great reluctance, I had to listen to my head and not my heart and call it a day.

'You can try it again next year,' Tim had told me trying to raise my spirits after I called him in tears to tell him the attempt was over. I knew quitting was the right thing to do but I still felt completely dejected and disappointed. I hated having to give up on something I had worked so hard towards accomplishing because one muscle had let me down.

After giving myself time to recover and regroup, I knew I had to try again. I set my sights on doing it the following year, and this time I was determined to finish. I had learnt a lot from the aborted attempt and I knew in order to succeed the second time, I had to get the logistics and crew right and start the run injury-free. Starting in Scotland rather than Cornwall would give me a fresh start. I am a great believer in positive thinking so told myself this was a new attempt, and this time nothing was going to stop me. But once again it seemed luck was not on my side. Three weeks before the record attempt was due to start, I was involved in a collision with another car while driving to the shops. My vehicle was struck head-on by another car and I suffered from whiplash due to the impact. It was touch-and-go whether I would be able to make the start line. But after seeing doctors and my osteopath, I was given the all-clear to proceed. The world record attempt was on.

What had happened the year before was in the back of my mind as I stepped out of the motorhome in John o'Groats that July morning, feeling full of adrenaline. I didn't want to fail again. I headed to the campsite entrance where my journey would begin on the same spot as many others had started their own JOGLE quests (or finished them). A giant white line was marked out on the road with the words 'START' and 'FINISH' emblazoned on either side in capital letters, enabling the words to be read depending on the direction you approached from. Our early start meant there were few people around so there was none of the gravitas or excitement I had experienced at the beginning of other races. There was no jostling for the best position on the start, as mine was the only foot toeing the line, poised and ready for the crew to tell me to begin. Becky was ready to mount her bike to cycle behind me and Alan was beside the line stopwatch in hand ready to start the clock on my record attempt. Meanwhile, Karyn and Phil sought witnesses to confirm the time they had seen me leave.

I took a deep breath as Alan shouted: 'Three, two, one, GO!' and then I was off on my epic journey to run the length of Britain. As I began to run my heart was pounding as I contemplated just how big the adventure I was embarking on was. While Becky tailed me on the bike, the others remained to pack up the motorhomes – which were adorned with the details of my world record attempt, including the logos of two businesses that had sponsored me – ICG and Cazenove Capital and how to donate money to Beat, the UK's eating disorder charity, which I was raising money for. The first motorhome would drive ahead to my first four-hour stop while the other would leapfrog me every two to three miles. To any people passing by when we were all on the move, we must have looked like something out of *The Wacky Races*, with me as Penelope Pitstop at the front decked out in pink.

After all the planning and preparation, it was a relief to finally get going and leave John o'Groats behind. Arriving there the night before had been a bit of an anti-climax. It was grey, drizzly and desolate with a derelict hotel perched on the cliff adding to the feeling that this was a place the world had long ago forgotten. The spot where we had set up camp had seemed isolated but, true to form, Karyn had met other people on the site when she had been out and about who were all there for similar reasons to me – one runner was also planning to run to Land's End, a group intended to cycle and one lady was walking the distance in memory of her late mother. Karyn had been fascinated by their motivation to do it and why the route was a rite of passage for so many. She had met a group of cyclists when heading to the toilet block before we set off on the first morning who were astonished by our plans.

'They said it took them nine days to cycle here from Land's End so they think it will be amazing if you'll manage it in less than 13 days' running,' she told me later.

It would be amazing if I could do it – and in all honesty, I didn't know if I would be able to manage it. But I was going to give it everything I had; failure wasn't an option this time.

I felt confident it was possible on that first morning as the opening miles flew by thanks to my fresh legs and the distraction of the spectacular Highland scenery around me. I began to relax into the run, feeling surprisingly perky. I was happy to finally be on my way after all the preparation and the previous year's disappointment. Completing the first ten miles running down a single lane from the campsite to join the A99 felt like a stroll in the park. It reminded me of how far I had come in the last ten years. When I was 36, I had barely been able to run for ten minutes, let alone ten miles. If you'd have told me then I would be attempting to run 840 miles and set a world record, I'd have thought you were completely mad.

Back then my motivation to run had not been to achieve records or win races, it had simply been because I wanted thinner legs. I was recovering from an eating disorder that had plagued my teens and twenties and while I'd had treatment to help me battle my demons and overcome my body dysmorphia, I still had a hang-up when it came to my legs. While some people have bad hair days, I had bad leg days. Those were the days when whatever I wore, or whatever angle I looked at them, I didn't think my legs looked good. They looked fat and ugly and I couldn't bear them.

I envied anyone who had thin legs. I thought theirs looked beautiful compared to mine, which I believed were big and wobbly, and I wondered how they got them. I found the answer when I was talking to another mother at the school gates one warm day as we were waiting to collect our children. I told her I wished I had better legs so I could get them out in the summer to wear dresses and shorts and feel more attractive. She recommended I try running as she had noticed a change in her own leg shape once she took up jogging.

That's it then, I thought. *The key to getting the lean legs I have always dreamed of is running.*

I was already a member of a gym where I joined in various exercise classes. I occasionally used some of the gym equipment but I had always been far too embarrassed to go on the treadmill. But now I had been told it could make my legs thinner, I was prepared to give it a try.

I felt ridiculous and self-conscious the first time I whirled the dreaded machine into action. I set the belt to turn as slowly as possible and attempted to jog. Even though the belt was going at a snail's pace I still struggled to keep up.

I was sure everyone was looking at me and judging how fit – or rather unfit – I was. I had barely been jogging for a minute when my heart started pounding and I was gasping for breath. I tried to keep going but I felt like I was going to have a heart attack.

I can't die at the gym, I thought, *for a start none of my family would know to look for me here when I don't come home.*

I desperately stopped the machine and stepped off defeated. As I bent over catching my breath, a muscular man took my place, putting me to shame as he upped the speed and ran at breakneck pace, bouncing in time with the belt and barely breaking a sweat. He made it look so easy.

At that moment, I could have easily given up and never gone back to the gym again. But as I watched this man on the treadmill, I was mesmerised by how marvellous his legs looked as they bounded back and forth in perfect sync with the whirling treadmill. His legs looked strong, toned and – best of all to me at that time – slim. If I could master running, I could have the legs of my dreams, I believed.

I kept going back three times a week, running on the treadmill with walking breaks in between and setting myself the goal to reach one mile running non-stop. Each time I went I tried to keep going for longer than the time before, even though I was still huffing and puffing and felt completely out of my depth.

Gradually it began to feel easier and after a few weeks my breathing became less laboured and my body seemed to be moving with slightly more finesse. I was elated on the day the distance marker ticked over to one mile after I had been running continuously. It may have only been a mile but I felt as though I had completed a marathon. I threw my arms in the air and whooped with joy, excitedly announcing to everyone in the gym, 'I just ran a MILE!' They were underwhelmed with my achievement and carried on their own workouts wondering what all the fuss was about, but I didn't care. It was the first goal I had set myself and the first goal I had achieved. I couldn't take the smile off my face for the rest of the day and it really spurred me on to set my next goal. Now I would try to run for two miles continuously, then three.

Once I hit the three-mile milestone I kept going back and running that distance every visit, gradually increasing my pace to see if I could complete the three miles in 24 minutes. I don't know why I picked that time but running faster seemed like a good idea as it meant my time on the treadmill would be over sooner, as I wasn't enjoying it. Those treadmill runs were boring and monotonous and I was only doing them because they were necessary. I had to stick with it as I was getting the results I wanted – when I looked in the mirror, I saw my legs were getting slimmer. That was all the motivation I needed to continue.

At that time, my three children, Emma, Ruaraidh (Rory) and Harri were aged 14, 12 and six, so going to the gym while they were at school had become something of a highlight of my day. It was a chance for me to get out of the house, meet other people and enjoy some 'me' time away from being a wife and mother.

It was still a very male-dominated domain back then, so there were few other women at the gym. This meant I soon started bumping into the same friendly faces every time I was in the changing rooms or heading to the treadmill. Initially we would say hello in passing, but as time went by, we found ourselves chatting about our lives and workouts. I learned that Maxine Ward (Max) and Louise Clamp were both mothers like me, although their children were younger than mine. They would leave their children in the crèche or at a playgroup so they could hit the gym. Like me, going to the gym was a chance for them to escape the pressures of motherhood for a short time, but, unlike me, they actually seemed to enjoy the exercise they did there. I thought Max was mad when she got to the gym with a big smile on her face and said she had been looking forward to her run all day. Yes, I enjoyed escaping the house, going to the gym and having a coffee there, but the actual exercise bit? I dreaded it. Running was not a pleasure but a chore, a means to an end to get the legs I wanted.

'It can be boring running on the treadmill all the time,' Max conceded when I moaned to her in the changing room about how little I had enjoyed my latest treadmill run.

'You should come and join us on our weekly run outside.'
Max and Louise said they met up with a group of friends
every week to run 10 miles along the Cuckoo Trail, an old
railway line in Sussex that has been converted into a trail path.

'Outside!' I exclaimed as if they had invited me to run on
the moon. 'Don't be silly. That's seven miles more than I
have run before and, well, it's outside!'

To me, running outside was an alien concept. It was the
1990s and running wasn't as popular as it is now. I only
considered running on the treadmill at the gym as an
acceptable place to run. The thought of running outside in
shorts and a T-shirt with my legs on show for all to see was
a scary and ridiculous idea.

'Don't worry, we'll stick to an easy pace and take a break
halfway,' Max replied, thinking my only concern was my
fitness. 'You'll love it!'

I wasn't convinced but Max and Louise were so
encouraging, their energy and enthusiasm was infectious.
How could I refuse?

It turns out they were right. From the moment the run
began, it was the best I had felt for a long time. It was a
perfect June day and the sun was shining through the trees
as we set off. There was a cool breeze and all I could see
was a picturesque route stretching out in front of me –
that certainly beat staring at the same wall when on the
treadmill. The minutes flew by as we ran past wild flowers
and under railway bridges, the hum of our chatter and the

pitter-patter of our feet mingling with the peaceful sound of birdsong.

This is glorious, I thought. *What have I been missing?*

The route was flat and pretty, the conversation flowed and before I knew it, we reached the halfway point and stopped for a break beside a small bridge.

'That's five miles done,' said Louise stopping her watch.

'Really? I have just run five miles?' I asked in disbelief. I couldn't believe it; it was the furthest I had ever run.

As we sipped water, one of the other ladies, Jan, who had joined us on a bike carrying a rucksack, pulled out snacks and started handing them around. At the prospect of eating, familiar alarm bells started ringing in my head. I instinctively thought about saying no when a banana was passed to me. I had plenty of well-used excuses for why I didn't need to eat at that moment – 'I'm not hungry', 'I had a big breakfast', 'I'll eat later'. But I remembered how weak I could feel when I didn't eat enough. I was already running low on energy from the first five miles of our run and I felt I was pushing my luck by wanting to do another five. I was enjoying the run so much, I didn't want to miss out because I didn't have the fuel to keep going. So I happily ate half the banana and for once I was grateful for the calories it provided. It might not seem like an accomplishment but to someone who had been battling an eating disorder for 15 years, it was a revelation. This was the start of me truly understanding that food wasn't the enemy but an essential part of helping me achieve my goals.

Refuelled and rested, we were ready to run again. I wondered as we set off back the way we had come if I would be able to manage another five miles but I truly surprised myself. We continued as before, the six of us running in sync and chatting away, greeting the dog walkers and cyclists we passed along the route.

Once again, the time flew by and we were soon only two miles from where we had started. I had been concerned that by the time I got to this point, I would be flagging and desperate to stop. But in fact I felt strong and was surprised by how much energy I still had. Without realising it, or making a conscious decision to do so, I suddenly started picking up the pace. I didn't say anything to the other girls but started pulling away from them as I got faster and faster.

I had never felt so free. It was like someone had given me a pair of wings and I could fly. I drove my arms and legs and kept getting quicker. I felt elated. My mind was clear. I forgot about the other girls running behind me, I forgot about my past, I forgot about being a mother and the jobs I would need to do when I got home. All that mattered was how I felt at that moment and all I thought about was how I was running. I kept pushing forward, willing myself on. *Should I slow down? No, keep going! Can I keep this pace up? Yes, I'm flying!*

For the first time in my life, I didn't hate my legs – I was delighted with them and what they were doing. It didn't matter what they looked like, it didn't matter how thin they were, what mattered was that they could keep going and keep me in this moment. They were no longer a source of anxiety but a wonderful mode of transport.

I felt so strong and empowered, no one could catch me. I kept running, sprinting to the end of the trail. When I reached the end, there was no one else around; the other girls weren't even in sight. I was amazed that I had managed to pull away from them by so much. I was also shocked I had managed to run a whole ten miles. I felt a massive sense of achievement – look at what I could do when I put my mind to it. The others caught up with me and were equally amazed by my turn of speed.

'Wow, you took off! Well done!' Max said with a smile. 'How did you feel?'

'Marvellous!' I replied. 'You were right! This beats the treadmill any day!'

We all clambered back into our cars to drive home and my legs were already starting to feel stiff and achy from my exertions. But even though I felt tired, I had never felt so exhilarated. I couldn't wait for the next opportunity to pull on my trainers again and go for another run in the great outdoors.

This is it, I thought. *I've found the secret to happiness.*

I continued to feel this 'runner's high' throughout the first day of my JOGLE challenge. As I made my way through the Highlands taking in the stunning views, running with ease, I knew how lucky I was to be there and how fortunate I was to be able to run. I ran along the A99 with lush, green hills off to my right and magnificent views of the North Sea, which was calm with gently rolling waves glistening in the summer sun, on my left. I was happy and healthy embarking on a grand adventure on two feet. We arrived in Tain on schedule and I was delighted to be able to tick off the first day without any hiccups. One down, 11 to go.

Day two: Tain to Kingussie, 75 miles

My good fortune continued as I set off on day two, which would involve running just over 75 miles to Kingussie, a Highland town within the breathtakingly beautiful Cairngorms National Park. My legs were a little heavy from the previous day's exertions but I was used to running back-to-back long runs in training, so my muscles soon warmed up and I relaxed into my running rhythm.

I was still relatively fresh (despite running 85 miles the day before) but making it to the next stopping point would be far from mentally or physically easy. Thinking about the whole day ahead was too much for my brain to cope with so each day I decided to focus on a certain landmark or a checkpoint to aim for to help me make it through. Sometimes I would just focus on reaching the next lamp post, the milestones didn't matter as long as they kept me moving towards Land's End.

Today's target was reaching the Kessock Bridge in Inverness, about halfway through my running day, as I knew my friends and family were waiting there to cheer me on.

As I got closer to the bridge, I was met by a family with two young children who had heard about my run and had wanted to come and wave me past as if it was a royal visit. They had timed it perfectly thanks to the fact I was wearing a GPS tracker that had been programmed into my mobile phone. At the time, this technology was mostly used to track people travelling in areas of risk around the world, not by runners. I believe I was one of the first to have the ability for people to follow me 'live'. I had set it up so friends, family and sponsors could follow my journey online in the form of a pink dot bobbing along a map. It was flattering to discover complete strangers were also logging on to follow and support me. It was a special moment when the two children declared they 'wanted to be like Mimi' and ran along beside me on the grass verge for a few metres.

My happiness continued as I stepped on to the kilometre-long cable-stayed Kessock Bridge, which majestically stretches across the Moray Firth. It was a marvellous feeling knowing that my friends and family were all further along waiting for me. As I drew closer to the waving and cheering group I saw they had decorated the bridge with pink balloons. I then heard another sound carried on the wind – bagpipes. My mother had arranged for a piper – Andy Venters – to play for me as I ran past them and as I got closer I recognised the tune: it was one that Andy had written for my father who had died the year before. The thought my father wouldn't be standing with my mother as I ran by brought a tear to my eye but as I got closer to the enthusiastic crowd, I couldn't feel sad for long. Seeing my mother and a large contingent of friends and family all there to greet me and wish me well was joyful and uplifting. I stopped for quick hugs, hellos and thank-yous before I was back running again with a beaming smile on my face. Seeing them spurred me on and gave me renewed energy for the miles ahead. The boosts from friendly faces didn't stop there. As I approached layby 178 near Daviot to stop for lunch (it was only when doing this run I discovered all laybys are numbered), I saw two people I recognised waiting for me.

That looks like Roddy and Caroline MacLeod, I thought. *What are they doing here?*

They were the parents of my friend Kate Edwards and I was touched they had made the huge effort to come and see me. We chatted for a while as I took a break to eat some sandwiches that had been lovingly prepared by my crew. Later the same day, I had another surprise visit from my long-standing friends Ann and Alistair who live in Balliefurth Farm, near Granton-on-Spey, which I passed close to on my route. I never expected people to make such an effort to see me and it really made a difference to how I felt. Enthusiastic, supportive race spectators should never underestimate the difference they can make in helping a runner keep going.

Day three: Kingussie to Inveralmond, 68 miles

I continued to make steady progress through Scotland, reaching Inveralmond to the north of Perth by the end of day three. The scariest moment of the day came when I ran over the Drumochter Summit – 1,516 feet above sea level. The sun had disappeared, replaced by a dark grey sky, and the rain started tipping it down. I felt as though all the rain had been saving itself up to be dumped on me as I ran along this treacherous section of the A9, where large lorries sped past soaking me with further spray. I was terrified they wouldn't be able to see me despite my accompanying crew and high-vis clothing. It was an immense relief when I made it to the other side of the summit unscathed.

Thanks to the tracker, friends and family continued to keep turning out to support me, the most memorable of which was when my godmother, Anne, and her husband, Neil, surprised me in Bruar. It was a very emotional encounter as I told her how the brooch she had given me as a baby had become a talisman and I never raced without it.

I was also attracting the attention of people who didn't know me as I ran through villages and towns and along main roads. One man got in touch via my website after seeing the address advertised on the motorhomes to tell me how he was flabbergasted to have seen me morning, noon and night – always running – as he had gone about his day. First of all he had seen me outside Kingussie near his home as he made his way to work. When he had travelled for a business meeting later near Pitlochry, he had seen me jogging along again. Then in the evening, he thought he must have been seeing things when he spotted me running by again as he went out for the evening in Perth with his wife. He couldn't believe I had been running all day and into the evening while they had continued their everyday tasks. They were both so impressed, they kindly made a donation to Beat.

Day four: Inveralmond to West Linton, 66 miles

Day four felt rather like a marvellous homecoming as I ran close to places where I had grown up. I had many friends and family in the area who kept popping up to cheer me on. Some even helped keep me going by running and cycling beside me. It was a wonderful day, full of support that proved I'd made the right decision to start the journey in my native Scotland.

There was one unwelcome visitor I could have done without though – I started suffering from a bout of cystitis, a common urinary tract infection. While the pain it gave me in my abdomen wasn't bad enough to stop me running, it was causing great discomfort as well as immense frustration. One of the symptoms of the condition is a constant need to pee. Yet often when you go, barely a drop comes out and you feel a burning, stinging sensation when trying to force yourself to pass the slightest bit of water. Having to keep needlessly stopping to use the motorhome loo, or to squat in a bush, wasted time I couldn't afford to lose when the world record was at stake. Becky thankfully managed to nip to a pharmacy to get me some medicine that eventually helped but it remained a painful nuisance until the treatment kicked in. It reminded me that even with the best-laid plans and all the training to prepare my body for the gruelling journey, there were still going to be unpredictable problems that could put my record attempt in jeopardy.

Day five: West Linton to Gretna Green, 65 miles

By now, the crew were working like clockwork in a slick routine to ensure we were on schedule, and as a result, they were getting as sleep-deprived as I was. Becky was always up at 4.20 a.m. to have my smoothie and a coffee ready to wake me up, and she made sure whoever was on cycling duty with me for the first shift was also up, fed and watered. Phil and Karyn were pitching in to do their crew duties with aplomb, while Alan would stay up late after I finished running close to midnight, to pore over the maps to check we were on the right route and work out what pace and mileage I would need to do the following day to stay on track. They were all united in the cause to get me up and running as and when I had to, as though I was a wind-up toy they would prep and then set on the road and watch me go. Such was their eye on the prize, when day five of the challenge fell on my 46th birthday, there was no time to celebrate when Becky woke me at 4.30 a.m. and handed me my trainers to pull on.

'Haven't I even got time to open a couple of cards?' I moaned as she cajoled me to get going.

'Not if you want to stay on track to get the record!' she told me. There was to be no slacking just because it was my birthday. So I set off running that day feeling rather sorry for myself and wondering why I had chosen to spend my birthday this way, rather than at a spa. However, this self-pity didn't last long – when I reached the first stopping point at 9 a.m. it was a wonderful surprise to find the motorhomes already there covered with pink balloons and inside a cupcake with a candle on waiting for me. Everyone pulled on party hats, handing one to me so I could wear it while I was allowed a 20-minute break to open cards and a few gifts. The crew had been keeping themselves entertained as they accompanied me for the past few days by seeing who could find the best item discarded on the roadside to give me as a present. I laughed as they presented me with their favourite finds – a scarf, a number of pens and a Tweetie Pie cuddly toy. Alan was particularly proud of his discovery – a pair of running tights – until on closer inspection we realised they were actually his! He had forgotten that he'd left them to dry on the back of one of the motorhomes after washing them and they had fallen off when the vehicle had driven ahead. After a chorus of 'Happy Birthday to You' (the first of many to make me smile throughout the day), I hit the road again with a spring in my step and a new mindset. Who needs a spa! I love running so what better way to spend my birthday. If I could achieve a world record thanks to my and my supportive crew's efforts, that would be the most marvellous present. I may have been a year older but I was getting better with age. I was much stronger and fitter than my 26- and 36-year-old self. By the end of day five, I'd covered 359 miles and been running for 88 hours and 58 minutes. I was feeling confident but I had to keep my head in check, as there was still a long way to go to reach Cornwall. I hadn't even made it out of Scotland yet.

CHAPTER TWO

BATTLING ANOREXIA AND LEARNING FOOD IS FUEL

Day six: Gretna Green to Kendal, 59 miles

Run, sleep, run, repeat. Run, sleep, run, repeat. This had become my daily routine and after nearly a week of this cycle, my body was starting to feel the toll. Getting out of bed was made easier on day six as I knew this was the day I would cross the border into England – a real psychological boost.

It was 5.30 a.m. when the significant moment arrived, but there wasn't much fanfare. The rest of the world was still sleeping and we were only half awake ourselves. Despite my fatigue, I felt buoyant. Making it from Scotland to England was a defining moment in the challenge and it made me feel invincible.

Way to go, Mimi, not far to go now, I thought to myself. Stupidly, I felt as though the record was in the bag now

I was nearly halfway. But as anyone who has ever run a long-distance race will know, getting to halfway is often the easy part and the second half is when you have to dig deep and hang on. I might have been on course for the record, but the second half of the race was going to be far from plain sailing.

Having got over the excitement of being in a new country, a few hours later we were beset by a delay. As I ran along the main road towards Carlisle, I started passing ominous signs warning 'ROAD AHEAD CLOSED', as the A74 was being converted into a motorway. The motorhomes would have to follow a diversion but Alan and I went on to speak to the workmen to see if there was any way we could squeeze through. After hearing about my world-record attempt, they kindly guided us through the construction area, showing us a footbridge that we could cross, enabling us to continue on a B road where we would eventually be reunited with the crew. It would be a slight detour but better than taking the long loop round the roadworks.

Entering into the north of England meant running through mountainous Cumbria. It was a stunning backdrop passing the peaks of the Lake District, but also somewhat dispiriting, as the hilly terrain meant my progress was slow. The effort of running up the steep inclines and declines as I followed the A6 through Shap and on to Kendal meant I had my lowest mileage day so far – only 59 miles. Some of the hills were so steep they felt as though they were vertical, so I was forced to reduce my pace and powerwalk instead of run up them. Luckily Alan had been giving me tips on how to walk briskly, as my main weakness was moving too slowly when I took a walking break, significantly reducing my average pace. Using his techniques, I managed to get my walking speed to 4 mph. However, the extra effort needed to tackle the hills was taking its toll on my feet, which were starting to ache and blisters were beginning to rub. I was also aware the longer it took me to reach our next destination the less sleep I would be able to get in order to stay within record time. The attempt was a constant juggling act of 'robbing Peter to pay Paul' in this way.

There was a welcome distraction to my low mood when we were joined on the A6 by a friend, Patrick Hobbs, who I had met during the Kalahari Augrabies Extreme Marathon in South Africa in 2006. He and his friend had spent the weekend at a car rally with their Marlin sports cars and came to see me on their way home, crossing our path about five miles south of Penrith in Hackthorpe. It was another gloriously sunny day and I was rather envious when they gave Karyn and Alan the chance to ride in the vintage cars with the roofs down, but it made me smile to see them enjoying the lift in such beautiful surroundings.

Later, another friend, Tim Welch, also brightened my otherwise demoralising day. He was an experienced ultrarunner I had met through racing and I was delighted when he decided to come and run with me for the second half of the day. Due to my pace slowing down, it took him longer than he expected to find us along the A6 and I tried to hide my despondency from him about how I was feeling when he arrived by giving him a big hug. As much as I loved the company of my crew, it was marvellous when anyone new joined me, even if they only ran with me for a few miles, as it gave me someone new to talk and listen to.

'You are your usual bright and lively self after six days of continuous running!' Tim observed. 'Anyone would think you were having a jolly day out in the country!'

My battered feet said otherwise.

'I think it is time you changed your trainers,' Phil advised me as I struggled to fit my swollen feet back into my shoes after a dinner break surrounded by fields of sheep en route to Kendal. We were fully prepared for the fact my feet would swell due to the high mileage and had packed trainers a size up for me to run in when this happened. What I hadn't accounted for was how the rest of my legs would also balloon, with one limb particularly engorged. The ankle joint was no longer visible, as my leg had become so puffy.

'Do you think you should see a doctor?' Karyn asked with concern.

'No, I'll get a massage from Becky later and just get on with it in the meantime,' I said. It wasn't preventing me from running, although I had developed a strange, limping running gait as a result. A doctor would have been bound to tell me the cure would be to stop running – and that wasn't an option. I was determined to soldier on – run, sleep, run, repeat.

I should really add 'eat' to this list as I was snacking constantly on the run and during breaks. I had one large meal a day and constantly grazed on food provided by my crew so I never felt hungry. They would ask what I would like at the next stop, and I would say 'surprise me,' my brain wasn't able to think about meals as well as running. So I left it to the crew to plan and prepare my food. Rather like I used to do for my children when they were young, at times they even had to spoon feed me so I could eat on the run or multitask on a rest break by having food and a massage at the same time. Handing control of what and when I ate over to the crew meant I didn't have to worry about my next meal or what it would be. It also meant I was less likely to hit an energy slump as I was constantly topped up with fuel. If left in my own hands, it would have been easy for me to delay eating till I felt hungry, or I could have forgotten to have a snack because I was so focused on just keeping going and getting to the next rest stop.

As it was, I have no recollection of ever feeling hungry during the entire challenge, as the crew did such a good job of feeding me – even though at the time I didn't always appreciate it. At one stage Becky joined me as I ran and handed me a bowl of chicken, carrots and pasta she had made on the motorhome stove. I took one mouthful and spat it out like a petulant toddler.

'Ewww, I don't like carrots! I'm not eating that!' I said, shoving the bowl back at her. I'm lucky I didn't end up wearing it. Becky kept her cool as I kept on running. Shortly after she caught up with me again, with the bowl in her hand.

'I have taken out the carrots and added some extra chicken so you are going to eat it,' she told me like a stern mother. 'If we all have to stop and wait for you to eat, then we will, as you are not taking another step until it's eaten. So eat!'

I sighed in defeat and gobbled it down as I knew Becky was right. Not eating now could cause me to run out of energy further down the line, which could cost me the record. Just as a car will stop functioning if it runs out of petrol, my body would stop running if it ran out of fuel from food. The snacks and meals given to me were all high in carbs and sugar to give me energy, plus some protein to aid muscle repair. Breakfast at 4.30 a.m. would be coffee with a fruit smoothie, then 'second breakfast' at around 9 a.m. would be porridge with honey or strawberry jam, sometimes with some fruit. Lunch would usually be a sandwich of some description as it was easy to prepare or take away if the crew passed a shop. In the evening, I'd have chicken or beef with potatoes or rice and a yoghurt for pudding. In between I would munch on snacks such as bananas, grapes, cheese and oatcakes, Jelly Babies, Twiglets, nuts, crisps and cake.

This constant consumption was in stark contrast to the eating habits of my youth. My teenage self would have been appalled and terrified by the amounts I was packing away for fear I'd get fat. Back then, I would often get by eating just an apple all day – and that would have been peeled to within an inch of its life first. I spent more than 15 years of my life suffering with anorexia, a secret and awful illness that got hold of me so tight, I struggled for years to let it go. Not only did it make me thin and frail, it turned me into a liar with absolutely no body confidence and no hope. The eating disorder took hold when I went to boarding school but the seeds had been sown earlier in my childhood when my parents unwittingly hired the nanny from hell. I don't know why but as soon as she arrived she took an instant dislike to me, and expressed her feelings with malice and violence for the two years she was in my life. My younger sister, Jacqui, and I lived in fear of when she would strike, as there seemed to be no rhyme or reason to any of it.

'You are a horrible, nasty girl,' she would say to me, often accompanied by kicking me in the thighs.

At the time, my father was a colonel in the British Army and we were living in Norway where he had been posted working with NATO. His job meant he was extremely busy, and, as an army wife, my mother had to support him doing various duties, which often involved going to day and evening functions. They hired a nanny to live with us and care for Jacqui and me. We'd had nannies before, nannies we had loved and had fun with – but this one was different.

I can't remember the first day she arrived. I just remember going from being a happy, carefree and confident six-year-old to one who was often scared and confused. The days when she would kick me and insult me were bad but the nights were so much worse. Every night while my little sister slept soundly in the bed next to mine, I would lie awake cowering under the covers in fear.

I would curl up on my side, one ear buried in my pillow, my soft toy dog pressed as hard as I could over the other. I would desperately try to block out the sound of *that woman* – which is now the only way I refer to her – approaching. A bogeyman coming to get you is the stuff of all childhood nightmares but for me, it was real.

The sound I dreaded would start to echo down the hallway. The heavy footfall of her steps along the floorboards towards our room. *Thump, thump, thump*. I would close my eyes and press the toy even harder against my ear, willing the sound to be in my imagination – but it would only get louder. The door would creak open and she'd loom above me. Before I even opened my eyes, I could sense her towering over me, her large, fat frame filling the room. She'd whip the covers off me and grab my wrist with her firm, chubby hand and drag me out of bed.

'You are a nasty little girl and you must be punished,' she'd hiss.

Most nights she would drag me to her room and shove me to the bottom of her single bed. 'You must stay there so I can make sure you don't get into any more trouble,' she ordered. She would then heave herself into the bed and sit up against the headboard reading a book as if nothing untoward had happened. I was treated like a dog that must sleep at her feet, although I often thought she would treat a dog better than she treated me – an innocent child she was meant to be caring for and protecting. I don't know how she could have been so cruel.

I would never know what horrors would be in store for me at her hands once she took me to her bedroom. My only hope was to try to sleep so I could block out what was happening. But often she would torture me by forcing me to stay awake. If I looked as though I was about to nod off as I lay huddled at the bottom of the bed, she would kick out with her legs, slamming her feet into my lower back or legs, causing me to wince in pain.

One night she had a particularly cruel idea. She turned the light from her reading lamp so it shone directly into my face. I instinctively screwed my eyes shut and tried to recoil away from the glare, but she just repositioned the lamp so it continued to dazzle me.

'What's the matter? Don't you like the light, Marina?' she sneered. 'Let's see if you like it when it's turned off.'

She then switched the lamp off. The room fell into darkness as a white haze hovered in front of my eyes from having to look directly at the bright light and I waited in fear of her next move.

Moments later, when the bulb had cooled, I could hear the sound of her unscrewing it from the socket. Panicked thoughts rushed around my head: *What's she up to? Why is this happening to me?* The next thing I knew, she grabbed my arm and pulled me to her. She took hold of my hand, pulled up my index finger and put it in her mouth, covering it with her saliva. I was both disgusted and terrified as her grip was firm on my small hand; it was completely trapped in her claws. She then kept her grip on my finger and pointed it towards the lamp. I could make out her round face framed by her dark hair in the dim light and see her lips curled into a cruel smile. Suddenly, she rammed my finger into the exposed light socket. I screamed out in agony as an electric shock jolted through my finger, burning my skin and causing a wave of pain through my body. She shoved my hand back to me saying, 'That'll teach you.'

Teach me what? What have I done wrong? I wondered as I cradled my hand to my chest. My finger was red, swollen and throbbing. I bit my lip, trying to suppress tears in case it merited a further punishment.

'And remember, don't you dare tell anyone about this, or I'll do the same thing to your little sister,' she warned me.

The next thing I remember is waking up in my own bed. As usual, I had no idea how I got back there. Jacqui was already awake and noticed my hand, which was red and swollen and starting to blister.

'What did she do?' she whispered in fear. I was terrified of the nanny, I couldn't begin to imagine how scared my younger sister was. I sobbed as I recalled the electric shock I had been given. Jacqui was horrified and gave me a hug but then a warning: 'You mustn't let Mummy and Daddy see your hand. If they find out, she'll kill us.'

The pair of us had lived in fear of this threat since we had moved to Norway, but there was no danger of the nanny's true self being revealed as she had my parents completely fooled. She was 19 years old and – to them – seemed like a sweet and responsible young woman. They had no idea what a monster she really was. In front of them, she was always sweetness and light. It was as if she had two personalities. Around my parents, she was a jolly, kind nanny who loved children and couldn't do enough for us. But then when we were alone with her, she was a cruel bully who continually told us how nasty, ugly and worthless we were. We kept quiet, as we were so afraid. We became adept at pretending to like her. My parents never saw evidence of the physical abuse she inflicted as whenever she attacked me, she would target my thighs and hips as they were areas always covered with clothes so my mother wouldn't spot any marks or bruises. That woman never kicked Jacqui in this way. Perhaps it was because she was younger and sweeter. I suppose it was also another way for her to control me, as she threatened that if I didn't take the beatings, she would do the same or worse to Jacqui. I had to stay quiet to protect her.

My hand injury would be more difficult to conceal but the nanny knew if I were challenged I would lie about how it happened; I was too scared of what she would do to either of us otherwise. So at the breakfast table that morning, I kept my hand hidden under the table as the nanny got out bowls and spoons for us to have cereal while my mother bustled around us getting ready to go out.

'Oooh, cornflakes, delicious,' she exclaimed as the nanny took the box out of the cupboard and began pouring them into our bowls.

'Oh yes, they do love their cornflakes, don't you, girls?' the nanny said in a kind voice she only used when my mother and father were present.

'Yes,' Jacqui and I replied meekly while exchanging a look that said otherwise. We hated cornflakes, or rather, we hated them the way they were served by that woman.

'Well, I'll see you later, girls,' my mother said giving Jacqui and me a kiss goodbye. 'I'll be back to have lunch with you.'

'Goodbye, we'll have a fun morning, see you later,' the nanny replied all smiles.

Then as soon as my mother was out the door, she reverted into her usual self.

'Here's some milk for your cereal I have saved especially for you two,' she said.

Not for the first time, she poured sour, gone-off milk into our bowls. The smell alone was enough to put us off eating but we were forced to swallow every last mouthful. She stood over us and wouldn't let us leave the breakfast table until we had clean bowls. They tasted revolting but Jacqui and I had no choice but to shovel the sour milk and soggy flakes into our mouths. I'd learned the best option was to eat as quickly as possible in the hope some of the disgusting flavour would bypass my taste buds. Is it any wonder that I later developed a revulsion to food and an eating disorder that could have killed me?

The nanny seemed to find any small way to inflict pain on us. When getting us dressed and doing our hair in the morning, she would pull the brush through my thick, blonde hair with such force, it yanked my head back.

'Ouch!' I'd complain with every brush stroke.

'Be quiet,' she'd snap. 'It's not my fault you are so ugly with such wiry, horrible hair. I have to brush it this hard to get the knots out.'

Like everything else, I had to accept it was my own fault, learn to bear it and suffer in silence.

She frequently found ways to needlessly scare us for her own amusement. For instance, she often told Jacqui and I never to swallow chewing gum – as if we did, it would wrap around our hearts and kill us. Then one day when Jacqui was chewing some, she came over and ordered her to swallow it. I will never forget the terror in my little sister's face as she refused.

'I can't! I'll die!' she'd wailed.

'Do it, or else!' the nanny had yelled at her, smirking with satisfaction when she saw how distressed Jacqui was as she complied by reluctantly swallowing the gum. Jacqui spent the rest of the afternoon convinced she was going to drop dead at any moment. The nanny took the cruel trick further by later playing dead herself. We found her slumped in a chair with an empty packet of chewing gum beside her.

'She's dead!' Jacqui said to me before the nanny sprung terrifyingly back to life with a roar.

'You stupid girls,' she said, undermining us as usual. 'You'll believe anything.'

On yet another frightening occasion, she could have been the death of Jacqui. She'd taken us for a walk along a river in Norway, which had frozen over due to the bitter cold of the winter months. Jacqui and I had a ball with us, which we had been happily playing with before the nanny seized it and kicked it across the ice.

'Well, go and get it back then!' she ordered my sister.

'I can't!' Jacqui replied. 'What if I fall through the ice?'

'Don't make her do it,' I pleaded. 'She could freeze to death if she falls in, and she can't swim.'

The nanny wouldn't budge and insisted Jacqui walk over the thin ice to retrieve the ball. I could barely breathe as I watched a terrified Jacqui tentatively step onto the frozen river and attempt to walk slowly towards the ball, the ice creaking and cracking beneath her feet. Sure enough, she had only gone a few steps when – *crack!* – the ice gave way completely and Jacqui fell into the icy water. She screamed in shock and flailed her arms in her desperate bid to stay afloat, causing more of the ice to break up around her and push her along the river as the current flowed. Watching it all unfold on the riverbank, I felt helpless.

'Do something!' I screamed at the nanny. 'You have to help her, she might drown!'

With absolutely no sense of urgency, the nanny reached Jacqui's position and held her leg over the water so Jacqui could grab on to it to pull herself out of the water. I rushed to help drag my sister back onto the bank, hugging her to try to give her back some warmth as she was shivering and soaked through. The nanny showed no comfort or concern. She just looked down on us and said: 'Don't tell anyone about this, or next time, I'll push you both in the river and you won't get out again.'

Once we got back to the house, she ran a bath so hot Jacqui yelped in pain when she was ordered to get into it. Even though it was boiling hot, that woman told her to 'just be quiet and get on with it'.

Eventually she inflicted an injury on me that couldn't be hidden and that was our salvation. It happened at bath time. After I'd got undressed, she'd frightened me so I started running scared around our large top-floor flat trying to avoid her clutches and having to be bathed by her. I ran from room to room, looking for somewhere to hide. In the end, I realised the only escape was to leave the house but as

I was naked, that wasn't an option. Trapped, I sat at the top of a flight of steep stairs going down from our apartment to our front door at the bottom, which led into a communal entrance hall.

This will have to do, I thought. *I'll wait here until Mummy gets home and then everything will be OK.*

But within minutes, the nanny had found me.

'You think you're safe, don't you?' she said menacingly.

She moved towards me and, before I could react, she took a few steps down the stairs, reaching for my ankles. She then pulled me down the staircase with all her might. My back and shoulders struck each rung and the carpet burned my skin as she dragged me down and down the staircase, all the way to the bottom as though I was a rag doll. I screamed and cried out in pain but she had no sympathy or remorse.

'This is your own fault, you nasty girl,' she said. She then grabbed my arm and yanked me back up the stairs again to throw me in the bath.

The following day, my mother was home in time to bathe us, which was such a wonderful treat for Jacqui and me. She was shocked when she noticed the red marks, grazes and bruises all down my back.

'What on earth has happened?' she asked me.

At first I was too scared to tell her the truth. I shook my head stubbornly and turned away so I didn't have to face her. But my refusal to confess only made her angry.

'Tell me how this happened right now,' she demanded. She started shouting at Jacqui. 'Do you know how this happened?' she yelled. 'One of you better tell me right now.'

We were both too scared of what the nanny would do to either of us if we spoke out, so we stayed tight-lipped while exchanging terrified glances. My mother became angrier and angrier, she shouted and even threatened to smack us unless we told her the truth. Jacqui and I were sobbing, we hated seeing our mother so mad. As the tension in the room escalated, Jacqui caved in.

'It was the nanny!' she cried out and my mother finally heard the terrible truth. She was stunned; she had no idea what had been going on under her roof. She sat down in shock and was horrified as I explained how the nanny had dragged me down the stairs the day before. She didn't need to hear any more and immediately took action. The nanny was sacked and kicked out of our home that night. We never saw her again. But while she was out of our lives, she remained in my head. Whenever I looked at myself in the mirror her words echoed around my head, *You're a nasty, horrible girl, why would anyone like you?*

I tried to banish all memories of the nanny from my mind and by the time I started at boarding school back in England, I couldn't have been happier. I made lots of friends and enjoyed all the activities and sport on offer. I entered puberty earlier than my peers, starting my first period at the age of ten, and my breasts started to develop faster than my classmates, which I found excruciatingly embarrassing. While they were still able to wear vests or crop tops, I had to start wearing ugly bras. Some of the girls found it amusing to taunt me for being 'tubby' and 'fat'. Up until that point, I was never concerned about my weight, in fact, I don't remember ever giving it much thought. At first, I ignored the mean girls and hoped they would get bored, but the comments and jibes continued. 'Fatty', 'Your skirt's too tight', 'Have you looked at yourself in the mirror lately, or are you too fat to fit in?' were just some of the remarks they would make if I passed them in the corridor. Eventually, I looked at myself in the mirror and thought perhaps what they were saying was true. Certainly, I wasn't skinny. I didn't think I was fat either – but what did I know? On top of all the times I had heard the nanny call me ugly and horrible, I began to think she must have been right – there must be something nasty about me that made people dislike me. I blamed my body and believed that to be happy and popular, I had to be thin. After all, the nanny had been a terrible person and she had been fat, while my mother was lovely and she was thin. I believed I would have to be thin in order to be liked.

This belief was further endorsed when a friend at school, who had always been larger than me, returned after one summer break having lost a huge amount of weight. She looked like a different person and was brimming in confidence. Her popularity soared and she was constantly complimented for what she had achieved. I wanted to be a thin person like her; I wanted to be popular, well-liked and admired.

At the age of 14, I put myself on my first ever diet. I cut out all second helpings and although I loved puddings, I knew they had to go – it would be a sacrifice worth making to shed the pounds.

I'll show them all I'm not fat, I thought. The determination that has served me so well in my running endeavours was strong in me even at that age, and once I set my mind to losing weight, there was no way I wasn't going to stick to my diet. For the next few months, I stuck to my plan and the weight began to drop off, but no one noticed and the comments continued – more dramatic action was required. Now it wasn't just second helpings and puddings that were out, it was pretty much everything. I cut my daily food intake so drastically, sometimes I would go for days without eating anything, surviving on just coffee or water. If my stomach rumbled and I got hunger pains, I told myself this was a good thing – as it meant I was becoming thinner.

We had set meal times in the canteen at boarding school and it became easy to avoid eating as I learned numerous tricks to feign interest in my food while not consuming any of it. I could push it around my plate as I chatted to friends and arrange it in such a way that the portion would magically appear smaller, even though I hadn't eaten a bite.

The canteen staff and teachers took no notice of what we were eating so often I could go up and only get a bowl of soup, as I discovered this was the easiest food to make 'disappear' just by constantly whirling my spoon round the bowl and occasionally spilling some. Often I would say it was too hot as an excuse to delay eating, then lunchtime would be over and – hey presto! – I would have to dash off to my lesson leaving it untouched.

Avoiding eating while with my family was more problematic. My mother is a real foodie and loved to cook for us so I had to start lying all the time in order to get out of eating. I hated lying to her but it was necessary. When she'd present me with her home cooking, I'd turn it down by saying I'd already eaten, or that I wasn't hungry, or I'd become fussy about a certain ingredient. Christmas was my idea of hell; it was an absolute nightmare. There was so much food around and while this enhanced the enjoyment of the festive season for others, it made me dread what should have been a happy time. If I did have to eat when in company, I would then swiftly excuse myself to go and throw it up to purge it from my body immediately.

Then I found another ally in my quest to stay slim – laxatives. If I did have to eat and there wasn't an opportunity to throw it up again, I could take them to ensure the food passed through my body as quickly as possible. Taking them became addictive and at one point, I was getting through two packs a day.

As well as stopping me from getting fat, abstaining from food gave me a sense of power I had never felt before. When the nanny abused me and the girls at school taunted me over my breast size, I felt powerless and out of control. By changing my eating habits, I felt I finally had a say in what was happening to my own body.

The less I ate the thinner I became, and friends and family began to notice. 'You've lost weight', 'Aren't you looking slimmer,' they would say. I took their comments on my weight loss as compliments and it spurred me on in achieving my goal to become thinner – which, to me, meant I was also becoming a nicer, more likeable person. Soon the comments came with more worried tones – 'You're looking very thin', 'You're a shadow of yourself', 'You've lost too much weight'. But I didn't hear the concern and remained flattered and felt accomplished.

By the age of 15, my weight had plummeted to just below six stone and while people constantly told me I looked thinner, I didn't really believe them as I was in the grip of body dysmorphia. When I looked in the mirror, I saw a fat girl staring back at me. I couldn't understand why people began to think my frail figure was a problem, as I still thought I was overweight.

By now the school had noticed my dramatic weight loss and so one day I was summoned to the headmistress's office.

'I've been sent a letter I think you should hear,' Mrs Webb told me. She then started reading aloud a letter that had been sent from a former pupil, who I had known when I was in my first year and she had been in the sixth form. She was writing from her hospital bed in Hong Kong where she was being fed by a drip and was fighting for her life as she weighed just over four stone due to anorexia.

'Something to think about,' the head said, looking firmly at me after she had finished reading the gut-wrenching news. I felt terrible for the author but I couldn't understand why her letter was being read to me. I wasn't like her I thought – I wasn't thin, I was fat, all the girls had told me so, why did she think this girl's eating disorder was relevant to me?

The head then told me I had a choice – either I started eating or I would be sent home, as the school couldn't cope with me. She said they would start putting food aside for me at the canteen, as this way they would know if I had collected it. The thought of eating a big meal appalled me so I said the only thing I would eat at lunch was an apple and an orange. It was agreed these would be set aside for me each day and there would be repercussions if I didn't eat them. Each day I would dutifully collect the fruit but I wasn't going to let them have one up on me. Just because I had collected it, didn't mean I had to eat it, so I would give it away or peel and pick at the fruit so much there was barely anything left of it to eat. Short of force-feeding, there wasn't much else the school could do as I was so stubborn. Besides, I didn't want their help, as I didn't see that I had a problem. My mother encountered the same antagonism whenever she tried to make me eat. It was the cause of many arguments between us. I was defiant and unreachable. I didn't understand she was trying to help me; instead, I felt she was working against me and my desire to be thin.

My immune system was low due to my starvation and I constantly caught coughs and colds. In the January of 1978, ahead of sitting my O levels in the summer, I caught glandular fever. I became increasingly ill and as my dorm was at the top of the boarding house, it became more and more difficult for staff to look after me. It was decided it would be best for my recovery if I were flown home to Edinburgh. I was so frail I had to be pushed through the airport in a wheelchair, as I didn't have the energy to move. It must have been a real shock for my mother to see her daughter wheeled out to meet her looking more like a dying old woman than a teenager with her whole life ahead of her.

Once I was home, I slept for a week. This was perhaps the only time I realised my way of life wasn't normal – it wasn't right to need so much sleep. But I put it down to the fact I was sick with glandular fever. Being ill with an eating disorder was still not something I accepted. On a visit to my doctor who knew my medical history, I was warned unless I started eating, I would have no chance of passing my O levels, as my brain needed to be fed in order to thrive. I didn't believe him, so to prove his point, he asked me to bring one of my revision books to my next appointment. I thought this was rather odd, but did as I was told, and returned with my biology text book, as this was a subject I felt I knew well. He asked me to open the book at any page and then read it. Once I had read the page, he took the book off me and we chatted for a few minutes before he asked me questions about the page I had just read. I felt a moment of panic as I tried to recall the contents of the page. My mind went blank; however hard I tried, I couldn't remember a thing.

'You need to start eating. If you continue to starve your body, you will in all probability fail your exams,' the doctor told me, handing me back my book.

Reeling in bewilderment from what had happened, I tried really hard to eat more as I revised and sat my exams but it was a real struggle. Despite the doctor's warning, I still wasn't prepared for my appalling results when they were revealed in August. I had failed everything except English Literature. I would have to resit the exams in November. I returned to school and was allowed to start my A levels alongside resitting my O levels. After a huge amount of work with extra hours of study and a massive effort to consume some food, however meagre, to feed my brain, I eventually managed to pass both my O and A levels, going on to get my first job as a receptionist/secretary in Edinburgh, where I moved in to a flat with three other people.

As an independent, young professional, it had never been easier to skip meals. I wouldn't have time to eat breakfast before I left for work, and then I would go for a walk or look round the shops at lunch instead of eating. With no one at home to cook for me or tell me to eat, I wouldn't bother with dinner. If I did arrange to go out with friends in the evening and they wanted to go to a restaurant, I'd drink huge quantities of water to fill my stomach, and then excuse myself to throw up halfway through the meal to purge my body of any food I had eaten, as well as taking laxatives later.

It was around this time I got together with Tim. He was three years older than me and training to be a lieutenant in the Army. I thought he was the most gorgeous man I had ever met. I had known him through friends since I was 15, but when we first met he had a girlfriend, so we started out just being friends. Over time, as his other relationship fizzled out and our friendship became closer, we both realised we wanted something more and became a couple. I couldn't have been happier. It felt wonderful to have someone who wasn't family who loved me. He made me feel special and attractive, something I had never felt before.

He was aware I had a difficult relationship with food but he couldn't understand it, indeed nor could I. I would often lie to him about what I had eaten and I was now a pro at making it seem as though I had eaten more of the food on my plate than I actually had. He also witnessed the blazing battles I had with my mother over my weight, so he didn't want to cause me further stress.

A year or so later when Tim left the Army, he was placed on a resettlement course in London and I decided to leave Edinburgh with him so we could move in together. Unfortunately, my father, who had very high morals and was a bit old-fashioned, didn't approve of us living together before we were married. He felt so strongly about it, he refused to visit us until we became engaged in 1984 when I was 22.

My mother was increasingly worried about my eating habits now I was living further away from her and she kept trying to make me see sense. I eventually agreed to see a psychiatrist just to get her off my back. Sitting in the waiting room at Maudsley Hospital in London awaiting my appointment, I felt extremely out of place. I wasn't mad, why was I here? After still waiting to be seen 15 minutes after my scheduled appointment, I was about to walk out when my name was called. When I walked into the room, the consultant took one look at me and greeted me by saying: 'Ah Marina, you must be bulimic.'

How could he diagnose me before even speaking to me? I plucked up all the courage I had to reply: 'Shall we start again? I'll walk out the door, knock, and come back in again.'

After hearing about my eating habits and fear of food, he diagnosed me with severe anorexia and sought to discover what may have caused it. At this time, I no longer had any recollection of the cruelty I had endured at the hands of the nanny, as my mind had boxed all the terrible memories away so I didn't have to deal with them. When the consultant asked if there was anything traumatic in my childhood that could have prompted my eating disorder, all I could recall was one time my father smacked me for being naughty. The consultant tried to blame everything on my father and suggested if I resolved my 'issues' with him, I could begin my recovery. I walked away from the appointment feeling lost and confused, and no closer to conquering anorexia. I had a great relationship with my father; I knew my eating disorder was nothing to do with him.

Life went on and there were happy times ahead. Tim and I married at St John's Church in Edinburgh on the 27 October 1984. I remember being so nervous beforehand, I chain smoked as I had my hair done to try to calm down. Then in the car on the way to the church, I was shaking so much my bouquet was rattling on my lap. My father, travelling with me, turned to me and said, 'Here's a tip to make you feel less nervous: just imagine as you walk down the aisle that everyone is naked.' I laughed, as this reminded me of my hen night when my friends had arranged a 'stripping vicar' to attend. He had stripped everything off except his socks, leaving us all in hysterics. Walking down the aisle to marry the most handsome man in the world, I had a smile like a Cheshire cat on my face and stifled a giggle at the idea the vicar marrying us would just be wearing his socks. All my nerves disappeared when I stood with Tim at the altar and we said our vows, celebrating afterwards with all our friends and family. It was an amazing and special day I will cherish and remember for ever.

Three months after our wedding, to my complete surprise, I discovered I was pregnant. I was stunned when I got a positive pregnancy test, which I had only taken when feeling unwell to rule it out. I never expected it to be the reason I felt so tired and nauseous. My periods had been non-existent for the past two years due to the fact I wasn't eating, and doctors had constantly told me it was unlikely I'd be able to become a mother – I assumed this was a scare tactic meant to encourage me to eat. A lack of ovulation is a common side effect of anorexia, as a restricted calorie intake can disrupt the hormones needed to make the menstrual cycle occur. The brain of someone with an eating disorder is working hard to keep that person alive with the limited fuel it is getting, so energy is diverted to where it is needed. It is as if the brain sends a signal to shut the reproductive system down telling it, *You're not needed right now. It is hard enough keeping one body alive, let alone sustaining new life.*

Falling pregnant was a complete and utter shock. Tim and I were still in our early twenties and hadn't even discussed having a family. We both knew we wanted children one day, but we hadn't anticipated it would be so soon into our marriage. Once the news sunk in, we were both delighted but my eating disorder added another dimension to my feelings about it. One part of me was ecstatic after being told I might never have children, but the other half was terrified. My biggest fear was gaining weight and being pregnant made this inevitable and unavoidable. But I knew I had to battle my fear and change my ways for the sake of my unborn child. For the first time in years, I stopped taking laxatives and washed them all down the sink. I tried to eat more and resisted the urge to throw up afterwards.

While for many pregnant women, their changing body gives them a sense of pride, I watched in horror and disgust as my boobs became bigger, my waist disappeared and my clothes got tighter. I had to keep fighting so hard not to try to do something about it by dieting, vomiting or taking laxatives – I kept telling myself my first priority was to my baby, she had to be safe.

Once my bump became more pronounced and it was obvious I was expecting rather than overweight, I started to feel more comfortable. I realised I wasn't fat, I was pregnant, and the two things are very different. I was able to relax and enjoy the rest of my pregnancy. Our daughter Emma was born in November 1985 weighing 8 lb 3 oz. It felt amazing and wonderful becoming a mother. I remember when everyone left the hospital room and I was alone with Emma for the first time I just couldn't stop gazing into her big eyes as she stared back at me. I couldn't believe this precious little bundle was mine.

As soon as Emma was born, my eating disorder returned. I felt I had to lose the weight I had gained during pregnancy as quickly as possible so it was back to skipping meals and taking laxatives. I loved being a mother and Tim and I were keen to give Emma a brother or sister so we started trying for another baby when she was a year old. I expected it to take a while, as I'd only had one period since Emma was born – if you can even call it a period as it lasted half a day – so you can imagine our surprise and delight when I discovered I was pregnant again within the first month we had started trying. Again, I put the baby first throughout the pregnancy, resisting my old ways. Ruaraidh was born in August 1987 by Caesarean section, weighing exactly the same as his sister – 8 lb 3 oz.

Once again, after I gave birth my eating disorder returned with a vengeance, as I was desperate to lose the weight I had gained while pregnant. I didn't start taking laxatives again but I slipped back into many of my old bad habits. I started skipping meals and avoiding food. As a stay-at-home mother, this was a lot easier than it had been in my school days. Running around after two young children and putting their needs first meant I often didn't have time to eat, even if I had wanted to. And this time around, I was actively encouraged and complimented about 'losing my baby weight'. Thanks to restricting my diet again, I was back in my pre-pregnancy jeans two weeks after giving birth and I was praised for this by some people.

'Wow, you have done well getting back into your old clothes so quickly,' they would say to me. This kind of pressure to 'snap back' into shape is felt by many mothers and for someone with an eating disorder, I felt as though I was being given a seal of approval to diet.

At breakfast, I would only have time to have a coffee while I prepared the children's food and fed them. At lunch, I wouldn't make anything for myself but would just pick at whatever they didn't eat of their meal. I'd keep going by drinking pints of water to fill my stomach. In the evening, after putting the children to bed, Tim and I would have supper but I would never eat off my own plate. If I did eat, I didn't like to see how much I was consuming so I preferred to graze on snacks – a titbit here, a bite of something there. I hated being presented with a large portion on a plate, as that would be undeniable evidence of how much I had eaten, and I couldn't face knowing that. So instead of having my own plate of food at supper time, I would just put a little extra of whatever we were eating onto Tim's plate and eat off that. I know now that seems absurd but at the time it was normal to me, and so sharing his plate became normal for Tim too. He hated it and would much rather I had my own plate of food but he never said anything, as he knew I wouldn't listen. He figured that at least if I was eating off his plate, I was eating something.

We were very sociable so this did prove to be a problem if we went to dinner parties or to restaurants with friends. I preferred to work around my eating issues than turn down an invitation or miss out on a special occasion. I would excuse myself as quickly as possible after eating so I could throw up in the loo. I always thought I was being discreet when I crept off to be sick but I'm sure they all knew what I was up to. I knew when invited to a dinner party that it wasn't very polite to bring up any food my host had spent time and money to prepare, so I overcompensated by being the life and soul of the party. I never wanted people to see the side of me who loathed her appearance and didn't have any body confidence so I was always bubbly, funny and game for a laugh. If people saw how happy and fun I was, they would never believe I could be suffering from an eating disorder.

Being sick after eating always made me feel instantly better about myself because I had an empty stomach. It was a feeling of relief and euphoria: I wasn't going to get fat. However, it was never a pleasant experience. It would take a huge amount of effort to force myself to vomit and my face and stomach would feel the strain. Part of me would be thinking, *I'm not going to be able to do this* while another told me, *You have to do this, you need to do it*, till eventually my efforts would pay off. While I felt content after managing to bring my food back up, I was always left with a revolting residue of sick in my mouth. It also brought the risk of another unfortunate side effect – rotten teeth. Throwing up food can bring up stomach acid, which can erode the tooth enamel, and when you are vomiting as much as I was, my teeth were in great danger of being destroyed. I believed the solution was to start carrying a toothbrush and toothpaste with me in my handbag everywhere I went, allowing me to brush my teeth after being sick. I have since been told it is not recommended to brush your teeth immediately after vomiting as it can cause further abrasion to tooth enamel. But at the time, it was another unusual habit that for me had become quite normal and part of my everyday life.

The weighing scales were another prominent part of my daily life. I was obsessed with my weight and would check it up to ten times a day to ensure it wasn't creeping up. Every time I stepped on to the device, I would be terrified there would be an increase. If there ever was, even if it was just by half a pound, I would be mortified. I would go over what I could have eaten to cause such an increase and punish myself by eating even less the following day. This was another way for me to try to take control over my life and my body. I wasn't trying to get to a goal weight and I wasn't as light as I had been in my school days but I was desperate to control the scales and ensure the measurement never went up. One day I weighed myself and the number rose by the tiniest of amounts. It didn't matter how much it had risen by, or that the measurement could have been effected by a number of other factors, to me, it spelled disaster. I had failed in ensuring I didn't gain weight and I was fat. The scales weren't showing me the lower figure I wanted to see, so I stamped up and down on them in anger and frustration. I stamped so hard, they actually broke. When I calmed down, I decided I wouldn't replace them. I knew it wasn't normal to weigh myself so many times a day and to get so worked up by the results. I was finally reaching the point of realising I needed help and I was aware this obsession with my weight wasn't doing me, or my family, any good. To this day, I continue to avoid being weighed, as I simply don't want to know. The figure on the scales is irrelevant to me now; health and happiness are far more important.

With the scales gone, I started to feel better as I was free of the constant need to check my weight and the fear that it may have increased. I started to consider the other elements of my lifestyle that were causing me distress. In the loo one day, trying to force myself to vomit again and feeling sore, frustrated and exhausted as a result, I finally began to question this behaviour and felt disgusted with myself.

Why are you doing this to yourself, Mimi? a voice in my head asked. Why was I making myself sick so often? Why was I always paranoid about every morsel I ate? Why couldn't I sit and eat supper with my husband using my own plate?

I realised I couldn't – and didn't want to – live like this any more. I wanted to be able to have a family meal, I wanted to enjoy eating out at a restaurant, I wanted to be happy. Most importantly of all, I didn't want my children to grow up thinking my behaviour was normal. I couldn't let them grow up thinking it was OK to be scared of food, to skip meals and to throw up everything they had eaten. Emma was now nearly three and Ruaraidh was 18 months old, so they were thankfully both still too young to be aware of my dangerous eating habits – but that wouldn't be the case for much longer. I needed to change for their sake. Being a mother was definitely what gave me the strength to at last acknowledge I had a problem. I realised I had to get better, not just for me, but for them. However, acknowledging I had a problem was only the first step on a very long and difficult road to overcoming this mental illness. Now I had to start allowing others to help me, and that wouldn't be easy.

I was back working part-time and I used the fact I was always busy to delay going to the doctor. I could always find a reason why it wasn't convenient to go. I realised if I couldn't bring myself to make an appointment, I would have to get someone else to do it for me. We had hired an au pair to look after the children during my working hours, so one morning, I asked if she would ring my doctor and arrange a time for me to go in. The appointment made, I summoned the courage to attend. But when I was there, I didn't know what to say. I sat in front of the doctor trying to find the right words. The tears rolled down my cheeks.

'Please help me or I might die,' I eventually sobbed.

I told him about my fear of food and how I either avoided it or threw it up to ensure I didn't put on weight and how I was terrified of being fat.

I was referred to St George's Hospital, Tooting, London, which was a leading clinic for people with eating disorders and other mental health problems. It took four months for me to get an appointment and during that time I continued to avoid eating as much as possible. Leaving my house to go to the first appointment I was full of mixed emotions. On one hand, it was exciting – these were my first steps on my road to recovery. But on the other hand, part of me still felt fearful that recovery equalled weight gain and a change in my body shape.

At my first appointment, I was petrified to learn one treatment plan would involve me being treated as an in-patient at the hospital. The idea of being away from home horrified me. I was needed as a wife and mother. I had two young children to look after, I couldn't be apart from them. Thankfully, the doctors agreed and it was decided it would be best for me to be treated as an out-patient rather than being admitted on to their hospital wards. I had to attend the clinic once a week for regular check-ups. Each time I had to be weighed, which I absolutely detested. They used the old-fashioned scales that had a balance bar at the back, with a slide that moved across the bar until it was balanced. I told the nurses I couldn't bear to know how much I weighed, so they let me stand on it backwards. Having been weighed, the remainder of the hour appointment was spent discussing my issues. They gave me an eating plan that they said I must stick to and I had to keep a record of everything I ate. The eating plan was a shocking read – how could they expect me to eat so much?

I had to eat 3,000 calories a day – the average recommended intake for a woman was almost half of that. To go from barely eating anything to consuming these amounts was a colossal ask. This was in 1989 and I'm glad to hear treatment is very different today and patients are now advised to up their calorie count gradually, eventually getting to the stage where they can eat three meals a day. The eating plan I was given then as an out-patient involved eating three set meals a day immediately, plus snacks on top of that. It seemed absurd when I was scared about eating anything at all to ask me to eat that much. I was to have porridge for breakfast; fruit and a biscuit as a morning snack; and not one but two rounds of sandwiches at lunch, along with a yoghurt. I was to have more fruit and a biscuit in the afternoon, then an evening meal of meat, potato and vegetables, which must always be followed with a pudding.

I wanted to get better but to go from one extreme to the other – from fasting to feasting – was impossible for me. I tried my best to stick to the plan but there wasn't a day I managed to eat everything recommended on the diet sheet. I knew I had to try so I resisted the urge to be sick as much as possible and I kept an honest diary of everything I ate, rather than lying and pretending I had eaten more.

However, the pressure to eat and the battle of wills in my head made me feel constantly stressed and anxious. I was now trapped in a desperate cycle. I knew I had to eat if I wanted to live but I was fighting against my entrenched belief that food was the enemy. Week after week I returned to the clinic to be weighed and attend the counselling session but it proved to be fruitless. Eight weeks after being given the eating plan, I was told I had actually lost more weight, not gained it. I was now back down to my lowest weight of just under six stone and my treatment had to be reassessed.

The doctors called Tim and me in for a meeting to explain my options. They said they had tried to treat me as an out-patient but unfortunately it wasn't working. Their next recommendation was to have me admitted to the specialist hospital as an in-patient. Both Tim and I were shocked and appalled by the idea. Hospitals were for sick people – and although I now knew I needed help, I still didn't class myself as that ill. I thought hospitals were for people dying from diseases like cancer, or needing life-saving treatment after being involved in accidents. I simply didn't see myself as in the same league as those unfortunate people. I wasn't aware then just how grave the situation can be for people with an eating disorder. I had no idea that eating disorders claim more lives than any other mental illness. One in five of those affected die prematurely as a result of the physical consequences or by suicide.

We did, however, agree to have a look around the unit, which only served to strengthen my resolve that this wasn't the path to recovery I wanted to go down. On our tour, I was shocked when I saw how thin and frail the other patients were. We were shown the rooms where people like me must stay when they are first admitted. It looked like a prison cell. There were bars over the windows to prevent patients from trying to throw food out. I was warned the staff knew all our tricks. They would search the beds to make sure food hadn't been hidden instead of eaten and if patients needed to go to the loo, a member of staff would take them there in a wheelchair, waiting outside with an ear to the door to ensure meals weren't being thrown up.

Exercise – and that included just walking yourself to the loo – was a privilege that had to be earned via weight gain. Imagine how that must feel. Only when you had reached your target weight and kept it on for a few weeks were you allowed to walk around and be let out of your 'cell' to stay in the main section of the hospital. Then it would take further weight gain to be allowed to be discharged to go home. Most patients were there for months.

I was allowed to go into one of the cells to chat to one of the young girls there. She was pleased to tell me that she had finally reached her target weight and as a result would soon be moved to the main ward, the next step forward in being allowed home. The fact she had reached her target weight surprised me, as I couldn't believe how skinny she still was.

'You are so thin,' I told her with motherly concern.

I was stunned by her reply: 'How can you say that? You are even thinner than I am.'

My body dysmorphia was still masking my true appearance from me. I was seeking help as I wanted to enhance my health and my lifestyle, but I still didn't acknowledge just how thin I was. Hearing how the young girl had been made to stay at the hospital until she gained weight was unbearable. I couldn't be away from my husband and children for so long. I had stopped eating as a means of taking some control of my life, but to be an in-patient here would mean I had come full circle and I would be powerless again. I knew the doctors and nurses had the patients' best interests at heart but it seemed a terrible way to live.

'You are not staying here,' said Tim, echoing my thoughts. *Hallelujah!* I thought with relief. At that moment, I couldn't have loved Tim more. He was on my side and we would get through this together.

But after this decision was made, I felt quite hopeless. Following an eating plan recommended by experts hadn't helped and being admitted to hospital seemed a horrible solution. But if they were my only options, how was I ever going to get better? I shared my fears with a friend, who had a difficult childhood in which she suffered sexual abuse. She told me of a hypnotist who helped her deal with her terrible past and recommended I give it a try. I was sceptical but I didn't have anything to lose so I decided to make an appointment.

The hypnotist specialised in helping people deal with traumatic past experiences and she told me the root of my eating disorder was bound to be something that happened in my childhood. If we could find out what it was, I would be better equipped to deal with it and move on. She explained how the brain can suppress particularly difficult memories and, over time, these become locked so far away, you don't remember them but they still influence your mood and behaviour. It turned out this was the case for me. All the memories I shared earlier about the nasty nanny were ones I only recalled under hypnosis. Until then, I had locked them away in part of my mind, as they were too terrible to think about or cope with. I had assumed my eating disorder had been sparked by the girls at school calling me names but that was merely a catalyst. It was the awful experiences with the nanny when I was so young that had really started it all.

I would lie on the hypnotist's couch and she would send me 'under', a feeling that's difficult to explain. My eyes would be closed and however hard I tried I couldn't open them. I would still be acutely aware of my other senses and could hear and think clearly. The hypnotist would ask me to visualise objects and then ask me to recall places from my childhood. When she asked me to visualise the bedroom I shared with my sister in Norway, I could never do it. All I could see was the nanny's bedroom and this would instantly create feelings of fear and loathing. I would start to cry and, as the hypnotist gently asked me why I was so sad, I would begin to remember the terrible things the nanny put me through. The emotions from that time which I hadn't felt for decades came flooding back – pain, confusion, fear and a desperate need to protect my sister.

I was only able to recall a selection of memories from that time. I know there must be many more from all the nights she took me to her bed – but I don't want to remember them. At times the hypnotist would try to push me to recall them but all I would see was the nanny's bedroom and patches of darkness. It was as if someone had gone through the images in my memory and censored them by covering them with black clouds and I couldn't see what was underneath. It seemed some of my memories were so unpleasant, my brain was working hard to prevent me reliving them.

I once remember reading how a survivor of the 1999 Paddington rail crash had experienced something similar. When she was pulled, badly injured and in shock, from the wreckage, she was hoisted above the tracks to safety, giving her a panoramic view of the carnage below. But years later, she said she couldn't recall the harrowing scenes she saw that day. She said her brain must have thought, *You have enough to take in, don't take this in too*, so she didn't. It must have been the same for me with those memories of the nanny. There was little to gain in reliving them and trying to recall those deeply buried memories became incredibly difficult and distressing, so the hypnotist stopped pushing me any further. Nonetheless, we now had an understanding of why my eating disorder took hold and enough information to help me deal with it. I was happy for any other memories to stay buried for ever.

With some of the memories of my childhood coming back, I was able to start talking to my parents and Jacqui about the time the nanny lived with us. It was something my mother had also wanted to forget. She felt such guilt that it had happened and blamed herself for not realising what was going on. I assured her I felt no anger or resentment towards her. It wasn't her fault and I have never blamed her. It was all the fault of that woman and I will never be able to understand why she acted the way she did towards me. As a mother, I know that children can be annoying and you can become exasperated if they misbehave, or you may be feeling ratty because they won't go to bed and you are sleep-deprived. But you should never react the way she did with violence and venom. I can only now imagine that something very bad must have happened to her in her own childhood to make her who she was. The way she treated me was meant in some twisted way to bolster her own fragile ego. I will never understand her behaviour and have struggled to find forgiveness, but finally I was beginning to make peace with it.

Recovering the memories about the nanny was a turning point in my recovery. I was facing my demons and confronting my fears. I began to realise that I was not, and never had been, a terrible person as she had led me to believe. It took time but I began to see that being fat didn't automatically make you a bad person, and being thin didn't instantly mean you were a nice one. I came to the realisation that what had happened to me was not my fault and hadn't happened because I was nasty and ugly.

I started learning to like myself and I realised how much the nanny had affected both my mental and physical health. She had made me feel worthless and out of control which had driven me to almost starve myself to death. I had spent decades of my life suffering because of her. I wasn't going to let her ruin the rest of my life. I was going to beat anorexia, it was not going to kill me, I wanted to live. With the support of my family, friends and professionals, I began to get better.

My relationship with food changed. I wasn't frightened of it any more and I knew eating wouldn't make me fat, ugly and unlovable. I still watched what I ate to an extent, as I wanted to eat a healthy, balanced diet, and I still wasn't, and never will be, one of those people who loved their food. I didn't savour flavours and textures or look forward to eating a particular dish. But I didn't actively avoid it at all costs any more either. Occasionally I would still throw up but rather than feel proud and content afterwards like I used to, I would feel disappointed and ask myself, 'Why did I do that?' The more a thought like that happened, the less frequent throwing up food became until I stopped doing it altogether. A big stepping stone in my recovery was the day I dished up supper for Tim and I – and I used two plates. It was a middle-sized plate rather than the normal-sized one Tim used but this was a huge deal and showed the progress I was making. I began to feel happier and healthier and I was ready to let go of the past and think about the future.

'How would you feel about having another baby?' I asked Tim as I approached my 30th birthday. He took some persuading but agreed and it didn't take long until I was pregnant again. Harri was born weighing 8 lb 9 oz and I felt totally different post-childbirth to my previous two pregnancies. This time I didn't feel anxious about losing the baby weight. I knew it would happen naturally over time, without me having to starve myself.

We moved out of London to Kent, meaning Tim would have to commute into the capital to carry on with his work as a financial consultant, but it was worth it to give our children more space to run around and enjoy the countryside. It was then I decided to join the gym to try to meet people and to get out of the house, as I was now a stay-at-home mother. My friends and family weren't concerned that I was a recovering anorexic seeking to exercise, as this had never been an element of my eating disorder. I had never been obsessed with burning calories via working out, I had only been consumed by not taking on any calories in the first place. I had tried to run once as a teenager, heading out early one morning on the roads surrounding my boarding school. I didn't get very far as I was so weak and unfit. Huffing and puffing, I laboured along, attempting to keep dragging one foot in front of the other. Then I heard a vehicle approaching, which soon drew level with me and then overtook.

'Morning,' said the driver and as I glanced over I was aghast to see it was the milkman doing the rounds on his milk float. As the slow-moving vehicle left me in its wake, I threw in the towel.

That's it, I can't even run faster than a milk float! I thought. *Running is not for me.*

Twenty years later, my motivation to go to the gym wasn't weight loss but to socialise, so this was not an issue in my recovery. In fact, joining the gym led to me discovering a love of running I never imagined I would ever have – and this passion for the sport was the final nail in the coffin of my anorexia, making it dead and buried. Yes, my motivation to run may have been related to a body hang-up I still had about my legs which stemmed from my eating disorder, but my love of running gave me another reason to live. I will never know if my eating disorder could have returned if I hadn't discovered running. As I loved to run and learned that I needed to eat well in order to run well, starving myself has never seemed a viable option since I took up the sport. When I started running longer distances, I found I would feel faint and light-headed if I didn't have enough to eat beforehand. I might not enjoy eating, but I did enjoy running, and I understood without the former, the latter couldn't happen. Eating was now necessary to me, which it had never been before.

As well as helping to change my attitude towards food, running also changed my body image. When I put on my running gear, I didn't care what I looked like or whether I was fat or thin. Wearing sporty clothing made me feel strong and empowered. I was an athlete. In my youth, I had never felt any love for my body but now I could finally appreciate it because it meant I could run.

When I stopped doing all my runs on the treadmill, I also stepped away from seeing my reflection while exercising. There were no mirrors on my off-road runs through the scenic Kent countryside. I could run free from the worry of what I looked like. Then when I started racing, my appearance became even more irrelevant. Beauty was no currency here; there were no prizes for who crossed the finishing line looking the prettiest. It was time, position and performance that mattered. What your body could do, not what your body looked like.

My first ever race was the Hastings Half Marathon. Adverts for it kept popping up everywhere I went and after Max and Louise signed up, they encouraged me to enter as well. I was warned the route was quite hilly so I started incorporating hill repetitions into my training. I didn't care what time I finished in but I was determined to make it round running the whole way, and that included on the uphill sections.

It was such a well-organised race, and I loved the atmosphere and the camaraderie between the runners. I also loved the support we got from the crowds who lined the streets to cheer us on. Tim and the children were waiting for me at the finish to cheer me across the line so, if I had a bad patch, I would focus on making it to them. Before the halfway point, one of the dreaded hills I had been warned about loomed before me but I dug in and strode to the top without stopping. The downhill was much easier and my legs starting whirling faster and faster like a cartoon character's as I sped to the bottom. I carried on striding out after the decline fed into a straight stretch of road. I felt strong and in control.

Now I am a proper runner, I thought as I was swept along with the other competitors stampeding round the course with our numbers pinned to our vests. I reached the home straight on the seafront and the finish line was in sight further along the promenade. However, my legs were now getting tired and it felt as though I was having one of those classic dreams – trying to run but not moving anywhere. I kept stepping forward but the finish line on the horizon didn't seem to be getting any closer. Finally I made it and off to one side I could see the children waving and Tim holding a camcorder to capture the momentous occasion of me finishing my first ever race. As he had been filming for so long waiting for me to come in, the battery chose that moment to die. I was actually quite pleased though, as my pride at crossing the finish line was somewhat dented when a race walker pipped me to the post. I was chuffed to bits to have finished in 1 hour 43 minutes but it was a little annoying to know someone else had managed to walk the same distance at the same pace. But none of that mattered when my medal was hung around my neck. I felt like an Olympic champion.

I had been truly bitten by the running bug. Instead of my mind being preoccupied with calorie counting and what I weighed, I became consumed by how I could improve and when I could do my next race. Tim joked that I had swapped one obsession for another but he was delighted that this one was making me happy instead of miserable. I was so glad I had discovered running and thanks to the sport, I would go on to travel the world and make many friends. Running enabled me to regain my confidence, discover an inner strength I never knew I had, and helped me conquer my eating disorder. It didn't just change my life, it saved it.

CHAPTER THREE

RACING THE MARATHON DES SABLES AS A NOVICE

Day seven: Kendal to Warrington, 62 miles

It was approaching midnight when I stumbled into the motorhome for a much-needed sleep at the end of day seven of JOGLE. Becky had been cycling alongside me in the dark as I had been running through Preston on to Wigan along the A6. Despite the late hour, we had been amazed at how much traffic had been on the roads. Drivers tooted their horns as they passed us by and we would wave back to acknowledge their encouragement. You couldn't miss us thanks to our high-vis jackets and flashing lights around our arms and ankles, while the accompanying motorhomes were brightly covered in the names of my sponsors and the details of the eating disorder charity Beat, who I was raising money for. I was constantly touched by the amount of people who would spot us as they drove or cycled past, pulling over to wish me well and give a donation.

Others purposefully went out of their way to support me as word of my world-record attempt spread via the ultrarunning community, as well as through a few local papers. As we passed through Lancaster that day, someone I had never met before, who had been following my pink dot as it made its way south, stood on the route waiting for me to pass so they could give me some home-made sausages produced at their farm. Then when my mp3 player died, a friend of a friend said their teenage son would be happy for me to borrow his for the rest of the challenge. They found us along the route to drop it off. It meant I would have to listen to a 15-year-old boy's taste in music, which was quite different to my own, but I couldn't have been more grateful to him for his generosity. Listening to music was really helping me get through some of the tough sections of the day.

These are just two examples of how friendly and supportive everyone I met was as I made my way steadily towards Land's End, it really gave me a massive boost and on occasions reduced me to tears with the kindness people showed.

I was becoming very aware that I didn't smell at all fragrant and I'm sure many may have regretted taking the time to stop and give me a pat on the back once they had a whiff of me. By now having a shower was taking up too much time and energy so I would shower every other day and wash with wet wipes in between. At the end of day seven, I had to brave the shower unit in the motorhome as I really didn't think I could stand the smell myself any longer but standing up and trying to manoeuvre to wash in such a small shower was incredibly difficult and painful. Instead I sat on the shower tray and let the water cascade down on me. Scrubbing my naked, swollen body I couldn't believe how odd it looked. I was normally a dress size 8, but I was now more like a size 14. It wasn't body dysmorphia this time making my body appear larger than it actually was; it was all the inflammation caused by the constant pounding on tarmac, as well as the lack of sleep between running marathon after marathon after marathon.

What have I done to myself? I thought.

It was quite scary seeing my body look so distorted – what if it stayed like this and never went back to normal? It was a frightening thought and I vowed to start wearing compression clothing as soon as I got out of the shower in the hope this would keep the swelling at bay. But there was a problem – I couldn't get out of the shower. I felt so weak and exhausted I didn't have the strength to pull myself back up onto my feet and there was little space to get myself into a position where I could haul myself up.

How embarrassing, I am going to be stuck here naked for ever, I thought. *I'll probably have to be rescued by the fire brigade. How awful to have my world-record dream end in a nude slump in a motorhome shower.*

I had visions of my bewildered crew scratching their heads wondering where I was when I was supposed to be up and running the next morning, and then imagined my mortification when they told people: 'Mimi's JOGLE challenge is over. No, it wasn't that she couldn't carry on running, it was that she couldn't get out of the shower.' How embarrassing!

With that in mind, I managed to find the last reserve of energy I had that day to turn my swollen body over and get onto all fours so I could get back on my feet, dry off and pull some clothes on. All I had to do next was stumble to my bed at the back of the van knowing I could then fall asleep as soon as my head hit the soft pillow.

Day eight: Warrington to Shrewsbury, 56 miles

The next morning, I didn't have a clue where we were and I had lost track of what day it was. I no longer measured time in days of the week, now it was all about the number of days into the challenge. The route had been planned in advance and I relied on the crew to navigate and map read each day. Every morning when I stepped out of the motorhome I felt like Doctor Who leaving his TARDIS, not always knowing exactly where I was. Some mornings we would be on a dual carriageway lay-by, other times a supermarket car park, or beside a field surrounded by spectacular countryside. It was always dark when I started and finished running which added to my disorientation.

'Today is my last day with you,' Karyn announced as she cycled alongside me as I ran that morning. This gave me some context – it must have been day eight. Karyn was only able to join me for the first week of the challenge as she had pre-booked a holiday with her family so it would soon be time for her to depart. As I looked at what she was wearing that day I could tell the time hadn't come soon enough as she had become just as sleep-deprived as I was.

'Did you know you have your tracksuit bottoms on back to front and odd shoes on?' I asked her with a giggle as I watched her uncoordinated shoes go round on the pedals.

'So I have,' she laughed only noticing her mismatched attire for the first time. She'd become so totally focused on my needs she hadn't even noticed her own.

'Thank you so much for everything you have done, you have been absolutely brilliant and I wouldn't have managed to get this far without you,' I said giving her a big hug when we reached the next stop and it was time to bid my friend farewell.

'Well, I am not going to miss nipping off to pee in the bushes to save using the motorhome loo, or being cooped up in such a small space studying a map trying to work out where in the country we are,' Karyn joked. 'But I am going to miss you all and it is going to be hard going back to the "real world". I have had such a crazy, fantastic time on the road with you, I have quite forgotten about everything else!'

I knew exactly what she meant. This is one of the reasons I love ultrarunning. For however long the event lasts, you are in your own little bubble where all that matters is focusing on getting to the next checkpoint and putting one foot in front of the other until you get there – or finish. You are constantly living in the moment, other problems, people and world events are pushed to one side. World War III could have broken out in the week since we set off from John o'Groats but neither I nor any of the crew would have known as we were so caught up in our own little world.

Karyn left us and I hit the road again with a sense of sadness that a member of the team had gone. Karyn had been great at distracting me from the pain of my aching muscles when I ran by telling me a story or asking me questions completely unrelated to running. Today, I certainly needed distracting as it was scorching hot and getting warmer as the sun rose higher in the clear, blue sky. During a quick massage in the motorhome on my next break, we put the radio on and the DJ informed us it was the hottest day of the year so far. Luckily I love running in the heat, although it is more energy zapping, I find it much more enjoyable than running in the rain. I was amused to hear a phone-in describing what listeners were doing to bask in the heat wave: 'I'm off to the beach with a good book!' 'I've set up a paddling pool for the kids in the garden!' 'I'm off to a beer garden after work!'

'Well, I don't think they'll get a call from anyone saying they're running 56 miles today,' I joked.

I resumed running as the temperature rose into the thirties, wearing a baseball cap to shield my face from the sun and consuming extra water to counter dehydration. In reality the heat was the least of my worries as the aches and pains I was now feeling were a greater distraction. I wasn't fazed by the rise in temperature as I had run in far hotter before.

'If I can run in the Sahara desert, I can cope with this,' I told myself whenever the thought *It's too hot* popped up in my mind.

Seven years earlier, I had taken part in the infamous Marathon des Sables (MDS) – a race held in the Sahara desert in Morocco that is 156 miles long, staged over a week and dubbed the 'toughest footrace on earth'. It was the first multi-stage ultra I had ever done and to say it was a baptism of fire is something of an understatement.

The crazy journey had begun when Max bounded over to see me in the gym one day brandishing a running magazine with a gleam in her eyes. She knew I had enjoyed taking part in the Hastings Half Marathon and that I was keen to do another event.

'I've found our next race,' she proclaimed showing me the article she'd read on the Marathon des Sables. 'We have to do it,' she said pointing to the pictures of athletes running across giant sand dunes carrying heavy backpacks against a cloudless blue sky. I flicked through the pages showing pictures of determined runners crossing vast expanses of sand with no shade in sight, decked out in sunglasses and legionnaire hats to help protect them from the blistering sun. While many of them posed for the cameras with a smile on their face, others looked absolutely exhausted and beaten, using walking sticks to drag themselves along. The images that really caught my eye were the ones showing horrendous blistered feet.

'Doesn't it look fun!' Max exclaimed.

I laughed and was about to tell her it was a ridiculous idea, but as I skim-read the article, I became sucked in to how exciting it looked. The runners tackling the sand dunes with their backpacks looked like real adventurers and the U-shaped campsite set up in the middle of the desert looked like nothing I had ever seen before. I tried to imagine what it would be like to wake up in such a place, pull on my backpack and just run. It felt like the ultimate freedom and so far removed from my ordinary life.

The article stated that the race was 156 miles in total, broken up into six stages ranging in length from a half-marathon to 52 miles, to be run over the course of seven days. Despite reading these figures, it didn't cross my mind how far this was to run – or how much pain it would entail. To make it even more difficult, competitors were required to run carrying their own gear for the duration of the race, meaning sleeping bags, clothes, food, medical supplies and anything else required must all be squeezed into one backpack – I couldn't imagine being capable of that given the change of outfits, make-up and jewellery I usually liked to travel with. I knew all of it would be well outside my comfort zone but all I could think was *What a challenge and an adventure*. I marvelled at the prospect of travelling somewhere so exotic without my family. Some will tut at this but I had barely even touched my own passport since getting married. If Tim and I ever travelled abroad, he took care of all the important documents while I was in charge of the children. So this would be the first opportunity I had to travel without relying on Tim, and without the children relying on me.

'Let's do it,' I said to Max's delight.

In order to take part, I realised the first big hurdle I would have to overcome was not training my body to be able to run that far, but getting Tim to agree to it. He would have to be willing to look after our three children, now aged 15, 13 and seven, while I was away for a total of 12 days, not to mention helping out while I spent hours training at weekends, as that was the only time Louise, Max and I would be able to train together as their children were younger than mine so they couldn't do long runs on week days.

There was also the cost to consider – race entry fees, flights and essential equipment. Before discussing it with Tim, I sent off for all the information so I would be armed with the knowledge I needed to help win him over. This was before the days of getting everything you needed from a website. We did have a home computer but Tim always told me to be 'careful' when I used it (cheek!). There was no fast broadband back then so I had to impatiently wait while the slow dial-up system connected to the very basic race website when our landline wasn't needed for a call. On the site, I had to register my interest in order to be sent a full race pack in the post. I was so excited as I flicked through the information booklet when it finally landed on our doormat, I was like a kid in a sweet shop. I still wasn't worried about the physical challenge and only saw it as a grand adventure. All I had to do was convince Tim it was a good idea. When he got home from work that day, I had supper prepared and was ready to ply him with wine.

'I need to talk to you later,' I told him when he walked through the door – he looked a little bit worried. After supper he took a deep breath and said, 'Well, we'd better have this talk then.'

I think he was concerned I was going to tell him something serious concerning our relationship or the children so he couldn't have looked more confused when I said, 'I want to talk to you about running in the Sahara...'

I gave him all the details of the race, and told him about the cost and how we intended to raise money for flights and entry fee via sponsorship. He didn't look convinced.

'I really want to do this but I'll need your support,' I pleaded. 'You'll have to look after the children when I go on long training runs and when I'm away for the race.'

He flicked through the information with an intrigued look on his face, looking wide-eyed at some of the images of runners camping in the desert and emitting a bemused 'huh' sound as he saw runners jogging over sand dunes with their backpacks. It was the sound someone would make if you told them you enjoyed the pain of having your legs waxed. After some consideration he said, 'OK, fine, you go and do this race.'

He seemed quite amused by the idea. It almost felt as though he was giving me a patronising pat on the head while thinking, *Let the wife do this and then it will be out of her system.* I could tell he wasn't convinced I would actually go through with it. He read all the information and said to me: 'You do realise what's involved? How will you cope camping in the desert? You know how much you like your make-up and hairdryer and nice soft bed. Not to mention the fact you've never run more than 13 miles before, how are you going to manage 156 in the desert?'

'I can do it,' I replied defiantly – but inside I knew he had a point. Would I be able to run in the desert? And was I capable of running that far?

My father was equally shocked when I told him. He produced a note I had written when I was a child in Norway. On it in different colours I had written line after line stating: *I hate camping. I hate camping. I hate camping.* Like Tim, he couldn't believe I was now volunteering to go on a camping trip. But their doubts spurred me on and made me even more determined. So what if I had never even raced a marathon before? So what if I didn't know if I could manage 26 miles, let alone 156? It may have been naive of me as a novice runner to think I could manage six back-to-back marathons in the desert – but I wouldn't know if I could do it unless I tried.

Max had also convinced Louise to take part and they were delighted when I called to say Tim had given me the green light.

'I'm entering us as a team right away,' she said, 'and I have thought of the perfect team name – let's call ourselves the Tuff Muthers!'

We embarked on the training with vigour and it helped that we were all working together towards the same goal, supporting and encouraging one another as the weeks flew by. We felt that in order to be prepared for such a huge distance, we needed to have at least one ultra-race under our belts to boost our confidence so we looked for a race to enter in the UK. We found the Thames Meander, a 54-mile race held annually in February following the path of the river from Reading to Walton-on-Thames. We each ran carrying a 12 kg backpack so we could get used to racing with the weight. It was supposed to prepare us for the MDS but in terms of the climate and the going underfoot, running through the soggy British countryside couldn't have been more different to running in the Sahara desert. It had been a particularly wet winter and much of the route had been flooded, which meant we were diverted off the course on various sections and had to use a map and compass to navigate our way to the finish. It was cold, it was wet, it was muddy, but, oh, it was so much fun. We ran as a group and finding our way along the revised route all added to the merriment. I hadn't laughed so much in ages.

However, as the race progressed it started to get harder. My back began to ache from carrying the 12-kg load and my feet were beginning to blister. By the 22-mile mark, I felt so tired and sore, I wondered if I would be able to finish. It made me realise how much of a challenge I had taken on. After 22 tiring miles, how was I going to be able to run another 22 miles that day? And then how on earth would I be able to run more than 100 more in the desert four months later? Max and Louise were also feeling the strain and we helped one another keep going. Working as a team helped me carry on, I didn't want to be the one who couldn't make it to the end. Eventually we reached the finish line around 12 hours after we had set off. Official times had not been recorded due to having to run off course but we didn't mind as the time was irrelevant to us, all that mattered was we had made it round. We hugged and congratulated one another before collapsing in a heap to take the weight off our tired feet. Although I was exhausted, I was on cloud nine. Like many long distance runners, I quickly forgot about the pain of the race and only thought about the positive elements. I had loved the challenge, the race atmosphere and running as a team with my friends. Most of all, I had loved the buzz of pushing myself to carry on when finishing seemed impossible and the euphoria at making it to the end. I was definitely won over by ultrarunning and I couldn't wait to do the MDS. The longest day there was a 52-mile run and I had proved I was capable of that. However, I now had experience of just how tough distance racing can be. I may have finished one 54-mile run, but in the MDS, I would have to do it again, along with another five equally challenging long runs, in much more severe and difficult conditions. Each of the six stages of the race had to be completed within certain time limits or you would be removed from the competition. The safety of all runners is paramount to the organisers, so if their on-course medical team deems someone too unfit to continue, they can pull them out for the benefit of their own health. I didn't want to go all that way and find I couldn't finish due to lack of fitness, or fail because I couldn't reach a checkpoint in time.

Louise and Max felt the same way, we knew in order to succeed, we would have to train harder and run for longer. Louise produced a training plan based on her knowledge of running, although limited, she knew far more than Max and me – and as it turned out, our plan was spot on. It wasn't easy to get information on the type of training we should be doing as there weren't many websites or forums to turn to, compared to the masses of information available online now. As far as we were aware, very few British women had done the MDS before, making it extremely difficult to get advice from a female perspective. We were also mindful that we would have to fit our training in around family life and childcare. Typically we ran 60–80 miles a week, including two long runs of 15–30 miles a week on consecutive days. We would also do a weekly speed session and an easy run of whatever distance we could do in the time we had available. Additionally, I'd go to the gym twice a week to do some strength and conditioning exercises. I'd occasionally run on the treadmill to get the miles in if conditions were bad outside. I'd always have one or two days off a week to rest my body and catch up on the usual boring jobs that needed doing around the house.

Living in Kent meant we were lucky to live near Camber Sands in Rye, so some of our training sessions were spent there running along the beach to simulate running on the sand. To acclimatise to the heat, we planned two warm weather training trips – afforded thanks to the generosity of Allied Dunbar, a British life assurance company, who agreed to sponsor our team. The first week was spent at Club La Santa in Lanzarote, as we were told it was one of the best training camps in Europe. The complex is a sporty person's haven: nestled in among the apartments and restaurants there's a running track, Olympic-size swimming pool, tennis courts and a gym among other facilities all at visitors' disposal. Exercise classes are laid on every day, all of which are free, and they stage races from half-marathons to aquathons which anyone can join in. Many elite athletes and triathletes go there for the excellent facilities and the surrounding lunar-like landscape that provides miles of cycling and running routes in the sunshine with little traffic to worry about. It seems we certainly didn't look like the typical Club La Santa guests when we turned up on our first night and went to have a drink in the bar dressed up in high heels and dresses with full make-up on and perfectly styled hair. We had arranged to meet one of the on-site personal trainers so he could give us a training plan for our week there. When this highly toned Adonis walked in wearing shorts, flip-flops and a tight T-shirt, it was obvious from the expression on his face what he thought of the three of us girls on a jolly.

'Are you the three ladies planning to run Marathon des Sables?' he asked in disbelief, looking us up and down in our glamorous outfits. You could tell he had written us off and was thinking, *These girls couldn't cope if they broke a nail, how are they going to run in the desert?*

But we proved to him that you shouldn't judge a book by its cover as, by the end of the week, he admitted we had much more grit and determination than he had first given us credit for.

'You ladies are as tough as any of the Ironmen I have worked out with,' he told us after our final training session together. It was a real confidence boost and we returned home with renewed zest for our training.

Our second week later in the year was spent in South Africa, where Louise owned a house. This trip was invaluable as not only did we escape a week of training in a cold and grey Britain, we were able to spend a lot of sessions running in the heat on sand, as well as running up Table Mountain wearing full-weight backpacks.

It wasn't an easy transition for Tim to adapt to living with me now I was obsessed with my training and MDS race plans. Sunday was my long run day and he really wasn't used to me not being around at the weekend. The first time I headed off for a long, wintry training run with Louise and Max at 6 a.m., I returned home cold, damp and tired at 2 p.m., Tim was nowhere to be seen. As I stuck my head in the fridge desperate to eat the entire contents, the children came running in all moaning that they were starving, as they hadn't had lunch. I knew how they felt. All I wanted was to eat and relax in a nice, hot bubble bath.

'Where's your father?' I asked them to get shrugs in reply. I found him pottering around the garden oblivious to the time and to the fact the children (and I) were famished. I had to have a super quick dip in the bath and then make and serve lunch for us all by myself – and I wasn't happy about it. To rub salt into the wound, I knew Louise and Max were both returning home to a delicious roast dinner prepared for them by their husbands.

'You said you would support me on this,' I complained to Tim after we had eaten. 'I can't spend all morning running and then come home to cook. It's not fair on me or the children. I need to refuel and rest after a long run.' (I had started to pick up runners' lingo too.) I carried on grumbling about it the following week when I met Louise and Max for our next long Sunday run and told them how envious I was that they would have lunch on the table for them when they got home.

Lo and behold, when I walked in the front door that day, Tim was in the kitchen with an apron on giving Gordon Ramsay a run for his money.

'I've run a hot bubble bath for you upstairs and lunch will be on the table in half an hour,' he informed me. 'But you'll have to make the gravy, as I don't know how to do that!'

What a difference a week makes! From then on, he was a whizz in the kitchen at weekends. He also helped out looking after Harri or picking up Emma and Ruaraidh from their social events so I could fit in my runs, go to the gym and have the two warm weather training trips. To do the MDS itself, I would be away from home for another 12 days so I arranged for my mother to come and stay so he didn't have to do all the childcare alone and would be able to fit in a fishing trip to Scotland he had planned before I entered the MDS.

The children themselves were pretty indifferent to my running. They admired what I was doing – as long as it didn't impact on their own lives. On more than one occasion, Emma had a typical teenage strop if I told her I wouldn't be able to drive or pick her up from a party because I would be away running and she would whine it 'wasn't fair'. But she never missed out, if Tim was ever unable to drop her off or pick her up, I would arrange for a friend to. Meanwhile, Harri's viewpoint is best summed up by an exchange we had one day on the school run when she asked me what I would be doing while she was in lessons all day. When I told her I was going for a 30-mile run, she replied incredulously: 'Running 30 miles! Why can't you just be like a normal mum and stay at home and bake cakes?'

While Tim and my family were bemused but supportive of what I was doing, others were critical. I remember the reaction from other mums and friends when I first mentioned being away from home for the race.

'I couldn't possibly be away from my babies for that long,' one told me. Another chimed in, 'Neither could I. My husband wouldn't have a clue how to look after my three. I would return to absolute chaos!' Others were stunned that I was voluntarily choosing to leave my family behind to do something so physically challenging and gruelling.

'If I had a week off motherhood, I'd spend it lying on the sand sunbathing, not running across it!' one joked and the other mothers at the school gates chuckled and nodded in agreement.

I must have seemed completely mad to them, especially as few women took part in ultras in those days, and of those who did most weren't mothers with young children.

However, it was perfectly acceptable for a man to do so if he was a father with little ones at home. We mothers are often made to feel guilty about taking time for ourselves but once I put my trainers on and go for a run, I have so much more energy when I get back and I am less grumpy – which pleases my whole family. I can handle the stress of life better and that in turn makes me a better mother.

Mothers (and indeed all women) should never be made to feel guilty about exercising, as it can do wonders for our health and self-esteem and sets a good example to children that being active is a normal, everyday activity. Over the years, I had learned to be more thick-skinned, so I didn't let any criticism bother me. I knew my children were being left in good hands and wouldn't be missing out on anything as a result of me going away. As for me being mad to take part in the MDS at all, I already knew that: it was part of the appeal and the more anyone tried to pour water on my fiery passion to do it the more determined it made me feel. Just as in the past when I had wanted to prove to those who called me fat that I could be thin, now I wanted to prove to everyone who thought I couldn't run 156 miles in the desert that I could.

As the week of the race approached, one of the hardest tasks was working out what to pack and how to fit it all into the backpack I would have to carry the whole way. A number of items were compulsory and I laid everything out on our bed before I packed to check it was all there. I reread the race information to ensure I wasn't breaking any rules by missing anything. Every competitor's bag would be checked before the race to ensure they had all the essential, and potentially life-saving, items in their rucksack. If a compulsory item was missing, a competitor could be given a time penalty or disqualified. The must-have items included a penknife, an antivenom pump, a compass, antiseptic, a head torch, safety pins, a lighter, and a sleeping bag – I had never taken a single of these items on a 'holiday' before. I cast a longing look at my make-up bag and hairdryer, which would be staying at home. In order to maintain some semblance of a presentable appearance, I had already been to have my eyelashes tinted, since I wouldn't be able to wear mascara, and I'd had my legs waxed as I wouldn't be carrying a razor to shave them. An amused Tim had observed that with all these beauty treatments, it was as though I was preparing to be a guest at a wedding rather than a race competitor, but it made me feel better about being without my home comforts for so long, even if it was a little vain.

I didn't need to pack water, as this would be supplied by the organisers during the race, but I would have to carry all the food I would need for the duration of the race. I knew I had to pack as lightly as possible so I opted for Pot Noodles, crushing the pots so they wouldn't take up as much room, peanuts and energy bars, as well as sachets of powdered electrolyte drinks that could be added to water for extra carbs. An extra indulgence was a few miniature bottles of brandy, which Max, Louise and I thought would make a luxurious treat when added to a hot chocolate to drink in our tent in the evenings.

I folded my clothing as neatly as possible so I could cram everything in to the minimal space in my bag. I had running shorts, T-shirts and long-sleeved tops, socks, sun hats and of course my trainers – which were half a size larger than I would normally wear as I had been warned my feet could swell in the heat. I had also tracked down and bought some green parachute silk so Max, Lou and I could make gaiters over our trainers by gluing the silk to the soles and then tying the ends around our ankles with an elastic band. We had been advised this was essential to stop any sand getting into our shoes, causing an unnecessary additional discomfort. Then there was one more item of clothing I had to fit into my bag that I'm sure most other runners wouldn't have packed nor deemed essential for a desert race – a sparkly purple mini-dress. I had spotted it in a high-street shop when shopping with Harri and thought it would be fun if Max, Louise and I could finish in style in the party dresses. Given we would have to carry them the entire journey when space in our bags was at a premium, it did seem a little frivolous so my solution was to cut the lining out of each dress to make them even lighter. I felt excited and full of nervous anticipation as I painstakingly transferred everything spread across the bed into the small backpack, which would be all I had in the world for a week.

'Are you ready to go?' Tim asked when he got home from work and found my bag packed ready for my departure, which wasn't until another few days' time. I detected a hint of surprise in his voice and I'm sure what he really meant was *So, you're really going to go through with this*. He may have been bemused that I was indeed off to camp and run 156 miles across the Sahara, but I could tell he was also proud of me. I was packed, I'd completed the training and was ready to jet off on my grand adventure, which was now only 48 hours away. But then came a phone call that threw all my plans into disarray. It was a call every parent dreads – your child's school ringing to tell you they are in trouble. Not due to bad behaviour or missed homework but because of an accident. I could barely breathe from shock and fear as I was told I needed to pick Ruaraidh up right away and take him to A & E as his arm was 'in a bad way'. He had been involved in a freak accident in which a classroom door had swung into his arm with such force, the handle had become embedded in his flesh. He'd been left with a gaping wound when his arm was wrenched free and needed urgent treatment. All thoughts of the MDS were banished from my mind as I dashed to school and picked up my son, who was by now in shock, to take him to hospital. I couldn't imagine the pain he must have been in. Once there, doctors told me Ruaraidh needed an operation to stitch his muscles and skin back together. As he lay in bed recovering afterwards, hooked up to machines, with his arm in bandages, he looked so vulnerable. I was meant to be flying to Morocco the next day but how could I leave my little boy like this?

'I need to call Max and Louise and tell them I'm not going. I can't leave now,' I told my mother who was with me at Ruaraidh's bedside. 'He needs me.'

'But what about all the training you have done, Mimi, and all the money that has been spent?' she replied. 'You have to go, you must go.'

Tim later told me he agreed with her and between them, they tried to convince me to stick to my plans. It was a heart-breaking decision and I wrestled over what to do for hours. It was like two strong resolves within me were at war. There was my desire to be a dedicated runner, which had driven me to put in hours and hours of training to prove I could do a desert ultra, and my maternal instinct, which wanted to protect and nurture and couldn't leave my son when he was in need. After much consideration and reassurance from doctors that Ruaraidh would be fine and was recovering well, I decided I would go. I knew I was leaving him in good hands and I didn't want everything I had worked towards for the past few months to have been in vain. I didn't want to let my teammates down or our sponsors who believed in us.

The decision made, I didn't have any more time to lose. I had to refocus on my travel plans, double- and triple-check I had packed everything I needed and then get to the airport on time. The past few days had been such a whirlwind of emotions, it was only when I finally stopped as I sat on the plane for take-off that I could take it all in. The magnitude of what had happened hit me with the force of a crashing wave and I burst into tears. I was still worried sick about Ruaraidh and felt terrible for leaving him. Max and Louise comforted me and reassured me he would be fine and I grew calmer as the flight went on. The decision had been made and there was no turning back now. I had to look forward and focus on what lay ahead – I was about to touchdown in Africa and embark on the adventure of a lifetime.

I hoped everything that could go wrong had gone wrong and I would now be able to make my first foray into the desert without further hitches. But on arrival at the hotel in the city of Ouarzazate, where we would stay the night before heading to the course, I started feeling unwell. Perhaps it was because my immune system was low due to the stress of the previous few days but I had managed to pick up a stomach bug and I couldn't keep any food or fluids down. After throwing up my breakfast, I wondered how I was going to be able to run with my energy reserves so low. But I tried not to wallow. I reminded myself I had trained hard to come this far and I wasn't going to pull out now. I just had to get on with it and do my best.

Many of the competitors were staying at the same hotel as us and a coach had been laid on to take everyone out to the race start, a six-hour drive away. We left the hustle and bustle of Ouarzazate behind and evidence of civilisation gradually fell away as the coach ploughed on through the sandy expanse. There was nothing but sand as far as the eye could see – which proved to be a huge problem when we pulled over for a toilet break. The men did what men do and sauntered off a few yards to stand facing away from us to relieve themselves. Meanwhile, the women all looked around us wondering where on earth were we going to go? There was nothing, no rock, no bush, no tree to hide behind in an attempt to try to retain a modicum of modesty. But there was the coach.

'Right, girls,' I said taking charge of the bewildered bladder-holding group. 'Let's just go behind the coach where the men can't see us.'

We all went round to the other side of the coach and got ourselves into the squat position in a row, trying to avoid eye contact with one another. Then, just as we were in full flow, another set of coaches ferrying runners to the start came whizzing past with faces pressed up to the glass looking amused and aghast at our line of exposed bottoms. It was embarrassing but we had to laugh.

'We're in the desert now, we'd better get used to it,' Louise said. She was right – there weren't going to be any toilet blocks or plush bathrooms in the middle of the desert. We would be doing our business in a hole in the ground for the next week – no one ever said ultrarunning was glamorous.

Back on the coach, we drove deeper into the sun-soaked sandy wilderness until we literally reached the end of the road and the tarmac became sand. The buses weren't able to go any further so we were transferred on to army trucks for the final leg of our journey into the middle of nowhere. There was standing room only, so it wasn't very comfortable, but it wasn't long until we reached the first campsite, where we found tents set up waiting for us. It was like landing on Tatooine, I half expected Luke Skywalker to step out from under a tarpaulin or see a droid roll past. We were assigned a tent number and told we would sleep in that numbered tent at every overnight stop, along with the same six tentmates. I was relieved I already knew Max and Louise but it wouldn't be long till the rest of our tentmates felt like old friends too – and by a strange coincidence one of them actually was. Graham Hedger, who I had met years ago through Tim, was also doing his first MDS (and to make it even harder, he was going to do it in fancy dress as a snake). What a small world we live in!

It is probably a stretch to call what we were assigned to sleep in a tent as it was really just a piece of stretched fabric pinned down on each side and propped up with wooden poles. It was pretty draughty and liable to be blown down in strong winds so we decided everyone would take it in turns to sleep in the middle of the tent, since those sleeping on the edges would be the most exposed to the wind. The first day into night was a taste of the extremes to come, unbearably hot when the sun shone and then cold and windy when darkness fell. It was like summer turned to winter with the flick of a switch when the light of the sun was turned off. On that first night, spirits in the camp were high and anticipation was in the air. Debates raged over what items should remain in backpacks and what should be left behind, decisions that could make or break you further down the line.

Snuggled into my sleeping bag and wriggling to find a comfortable position on the sand, I could see the stars shining brightly in the black sky and I couldn't quite believe I was finally here. As I fell asleep, I hoped Ruaraidh and everyone back at home were OK. I had no way of communicating with my family in the desert. The mobile I owned then was the size of a brick so there was no point carrying the extra weight when I wasn't going to get a signal anyway. Being cut off from the outside world had its advantages, as it meant I could fully immerse myself in the adventure that was to come, and relish every day, hour and minute, forgetting about anything else – my world was now the race.

The following morning we had the obligatory kit check, and it felt like it went on for ages, with a line of competitors snaking back to the tents as they waited their turn. When we reached the front, our packs were emptied, with a member of staff raising an eyebrow in bewilderment when he pulled out one of our sparkly dresses. After each of the essential items was checked off the list, our bags were repacked and then weighed to ensure they didn't exceed the 12-kg limit. Louise was mortified when she was told hers was 14 kg and even the staff were stunned by its weight, telling her to lose some of her 'unnecessary' kit (no doubt thinking about our mini-dresses). The excess weight was actually down to the fact Louise had packed far too much food as she had been worried about running out. She then faced a dilemma over what to keep and what to leave behind.

With our backpacks finally all given the seal of approval, we then prepared ourselves to run, which felt rather like we were getting ready to go into space. We wrapped our trainers up in the parachute silk, tying it round our ankles giving us the illusion of moon boots, pulled our legionnaire hats on and wrapped bandanas round our necks, ready to be pulled over our faces so we could breathe in the event of a sand storm. Our backpacks were heaved on like oxygen tanks and after lathering any exposed skin in sun cream, we were ready for lift off. I couldn't help but giggle when I saw how bizarre we all looked but it was worth sacrificing style and dignity in order to be comfortable.

As we headed to the start line, the atmosphere was buzzing. Seven hundred runners of all ages and nationalities assembled, and a helicopter poised to follow our progress hovered overhead. It was all hugely exciting and like nothing I had ever experienced before. Then a mad Frenchman climbed on top of a Range Rover to shout race instructions to us like an officer motivating the troops for a cavalry charge. It was Patrick Bauer; this entire event was his brainchild. In 1984, the concert promoter had decided to walk 200 miles alone across this expanse of desert and in doing so decided the rest of us were missing out on sharing the challenging experience. Two years later, he organised the first MDS involving 186 runners and it quickly established a reputation as the 'toughest foot race on earth', attracting runners from all over the globe to take it on. Now thousands of people take part, supported by a full contingent of medical staff at every checkpoint. The start list over the years has included Olympians like James Cracknell, world-renowned adventurers like Ranulph Fiennes – and in 2001, three ultrarunning novice mothers from Kent, who knew more about changing nappies than we did running through the desert.

'Here we go, Tuff Muthers!' I said to Max and Louise. We might not have been seasoned athletes but what we lacked in experience we made up for in good humour and optimism.

Sun-tanned Patrick jigged atop the Range Rover as he continued his rallying call, most of which we couldn't understand as it was in French, and then began a countdown we could understand... *Trois, deux, un... ALLEZ!* We were off. The crowd surged forward running into battle. Max, Louise and I were quickly enveloped by runners who overtook leaving us for dust, or in this case, sand. I couldn't believe the speed of some of them.

'Don't they realise there are 156 miles to go?' I asked, as we plodded at a gentle pace while others zoomed by. The field soon started to spread out and I could see a line of runners snaking through the sand ahead like a line of ants. While the elite athletes were quickly out of view, we started to overtake others who were already paying the price for a sprint start and were having to walk.

On this first day, we would have to run about 37 miles with regular checkpoints to grab water, which had been delivered via four-by-fours as no other vehicles could get access. Anyone who didn't make it to the checkpoints within the cut-off time would be pulled out of the race. 'Doc Trotters', as the large medical team were affectionately known, would drive along the course in Jeeps at the hottest part of the day to watch and monitor the competitors to ensure no one was ever in too much trouble. At each checkpoint there would be a Doc Trotter tent to patch up battered feet or give intravenous drips where necessary. This was also to be avoided if possible, as an IV would incur a time penalty, and potentially lead to a runner being disqualified. Even though I was still feeling sick, I was determined this wouldn't happen to me, being disqualified would have been more unbearable than the discomfort I was in.

The conditions were brutal. The soft sand gave way easily underfoot so it took twice as much energy to lift off for the next step. This quickly sapped my energy while the bright sun was relentless from dawn till dusk and the temperature soared to 50°C. There were no clouds and no shade to offer any respite from the heat and the glare.

It was hard to get into a running rhythm due to the shifting sands underfoot but Louise, Max and I stayed together and urged one another along. It was tiring but we didn't complain; this is what we had signed up for, and we knew it wasn't going to be easy. It wasn't all bad as the scenery around us was awe-inspiring. We still couldn't believe where we were. As we ran through desert valleys, wadis and over dried-up lake beds, I listened to songs from *The Lion King* on my mp3 player. As I crested one dune and saw an expanse of sand below gleaming in the sun, it felt as though someone had dropped me into the Disney movie and I was Simba surveying his kingdom. I was no longer sat on the sofa watching the film, I was in it, listening to 'Circle of Life' and thinking how the MDS runners were like the animals in the opening credits, rushing across the plains to the same place in the wilderness. They were after a glimpse of newborn baby Simba; we just wanted a rest and a drink.

Finally, we made it. Day one complete and I was exhausted but happy. I was still struggling to keep down any food due to the stomach bug but I was able to manage a carbohydrate drink. The three of us decided we had truly earned our hot chocolate with a dash of brandy before we went to sleep. We heated the water up using a Hexi stove, a lightweight steel frame which came with fuel tablets that could be ignited with a lighter. It was easy to carry and perfect for camping. While the alcoholic hot chocolate had seemed like a great idea back in Britain, I soon realised it was not the drink of choice for Sahara trekkers. I only managed a mouthful, as it tasted disgusting. I felt so dehydrated I couldn't stomach the sweet and rich flavour. All I craved was a tall, cold, glass of ice water. The closest I got to satisfying this craving was the first drink of water in the mornings. It wasn't ice cold but it was as cool as I was going to get all day – the rest of the water we would be given would always be lukewarm thanks to being left out in the sun. That first gulp of water every morning was so refreshing, at that moment I would take it over any fancy cocktail or expensive champagne.

The water for every competitor was strictly rationed so everyone – male or female, old or young – got exactly the same. Only having an allocated amount of water each day was tough but fair and it was a relief not to have to carry heavy bottles of it ourselves. We soon found out what a precious commodity it was; some would start to barter for other people's rations but few would be willing to give any up. If runners got really desperate, they were allowed to be given extra but this would incur a time penalty. We didn't want to risk this in case it meant we didn't make a checkpoint before the cut-off. We also drank our water sparingly so we had a little remaining each day to wash ourselves – a total luxury.

The second day was known as 'Dune Day'. It seemed no one around the camp would utter these words without a heavy tone of foreboding. I half expected a bolt of lightning to flash through the sky accompanied by a crack of thunder as soon as someone uttered the words, *Dune Day*. We would be running for around 20 miles over the dreaded dunes. But these were no ordinary dunes: they were among the highest in the world, with some up to 500 ft tall. I was concerned by just how many of these we would face, as they were described as 'fields' of dunes. Fields! The dunes of day one had been tough enough, and now we would be tackling mountainous ones that covered acres of land. My quads ached just thinking about it.

Setting off on day two, we could see the dunes looming majestically ahead. As we got closer I was astounded by just how high they were; I felt like a tiny ant beside them. We found it impossible to run up the steep slopes and at times it felt like you were taking one step forward and two steps back as the sand would shift underfoot and send you sliding back down. It was then we remembered we'd packed walking poles and they proved invaluable for heaving us up and over dune after dune. It was hard, thirsty work but the view from the top of each dune was spectacular. I could see the other competitors stretching out far ahead and behind us in a thin line going up and down each dune like carriages on a big dipper rollercoaster.

We made it to the interim checkpoint before heading out into the main section of dunes. While we waited in a queue for water, the sun beat down on our heads and the atmosphere among the competitors was one of excitement mixed with a few nerves. Once at the front of the queue, each of us was only given 500 ml of water. Even the four-by-fours couldn't access this section of the desert so only a small number of bottles could be dropped off via helicopter. This ration would have to last us until the main checkpoint on the other side of the giant dunes.

'Let's plough on then, Tuff Muthers!' Louise said as she took a few sips of her refreshing ration. 'The sooner we finish the sooner we get more water.'

We continued to crest yet more tall dunes as the sun beat down on us and my quads and hamstrings were competing for which felt worse. We were finally given some brief respite as the route flattened out and we hoped it would be a nice, flat run in to the campsite. However, at the end of the day there was a cruel twist in the tail – yet more dunes. These were not as high as before but some were over two miles long and very steep. Where possible, we tried to go round rather than over them. It was such hard work. I had to keep telling myself over and over that the camp was going to be after the next dune. There were a number of such sandy red herrings before finally we did reach the last one and as we reached the peak, we could see the campsite beyond, a true oasis in the desert. We hardly had the energy to speak to one another that night, as all we wanted to do was kick off our trainers, inspect our blisters, cook our food and go to sleep. We all agreed Dune Day had been amazing but those mountains of sand were both beautiful and beastly.

Day three was supposed to be easy – if you can ever call running 24 miles across the Sahara easy. I was amazed at how much the landscape changed throughout the course. At times there would be seemingly never-ending stretches of sand, then we would run on the hard ground of dried-up riverbeds. Others sections were rocky underfoot causing shots of pain through the ball of your foot and ankle if you landed on a jagged one. At some points, we even had to do a spot of rock climbing and haul ourselves up and back down jagged tors. On these sections, everyone helped each other along, offering a hand to clamber over rocks, or pointing out the best spot for sure footing. It all added to the camaraderie and a feeling that we were all in it together, rather than race rivals.

For me, the worst part wasn't the climbing but the stretches where we ran through the wadis. Dropping down into the barren basin you could feel the heat even more intensely, as the sun shone down like a magnifying glass was being held above us to concentrate the rays on our backs. When you run in the heat, your body has to work harder to regulate your temperature by sweating to ensure you don't overheat. My body wasn't just working hard now, it was working overtime. As soon as I produced sweat, the liquid evaporated in the heat before it could cool me down, causing me to sweat even more and repeat the useless cycle. My shorts were stained with salt marks from the dried-up sweat and every orifice of my body – nose, eyes, mouth – felt completely parched and void of any fluid. On top of this, my illness was starting to take its toll. I still couldn't keep food down and I was suffering from bouts of diarrhoea. I assumed this was all part and parcel of the event so I wasn't duly concerned and thought I would just have to soldier on, but my pace was getting slower and slower. Max, Louise and I had vowed to run the whole race together so they slowed their pace to match mine. This made me feel even worse, they would be out of the heat and in the shade of the campsite much faster if I wasn't holding them up. They were amazing and didn't mind in the slightest. Louise gave me one of her energy gels at the next checkpoint which I could stomach and it really perked me up. They also graciously divided some of my non-compulsory kit between them to lighten my load, which made a massive difference. If you want to find out who your friends are, do a desert ultra with them.

I don't know how, but eventually we reached the campsite. I felt so drained and depleted, all I wanted to do was go and lie down in our tent and rest. But before we could get there, we were called over by some of the race officials and told we were to have a random spot check on our backpacks to ensure we were all still carrying the compulsory kit. As they unpacked my rucksack, checking off the essential items one by one, I had a horrible thought. I had lent my lighter to a campmate the night before and now couldn't remember if they had given it back to me. The official kept rummaging through my bag and I felt as anxious as a drug smuggler having their bag searched by customs. If my lighter wasn't there, I would be given a time penalty. I heaved a sigh of relief when he rummaged deep into the corner of my bag and found the lighter tucked away there.

'That's fine,' he said, dismissing me as he moved on to check Max and Louise were also carrying their compulsory items. Once all our bags were given the seal of approval, we stumbled back to our tents, wincing in pain as we took off our trainers. My feet were sore and blistered. I wasn't grateful to whoever had recommended wearing shoes half a size bigger than needed. My feet hadn't swelled that much and as a result I had rubbed blisters due to my feet sliding around in the oversized shoes, as well as making me feel as though I was running in clown shoes.

'I'd have been much better off with trainers my usual size,' I said.

'Me too,' Max agreed and she turned to show me her feet which were in an even worse state than mine. Her toenails were falling off and the red and angry sole of her foot looked like one giant blister.

'I think you two should get those feet seen to,' Louise told us; somehow she had miraculously managed to survive the past three days with barely any chafing.

I didn't like the idea of the Doc Trotters tending to my blisters as I had heard horror stories of how they ruthlessly cut them completely off the soles of people's feet. I didn't want that to happen to me, as it sounded far too painful. But it would be useful to use their water to wash our feet instead of our own rations, so we hobbled to the medical tent to find ourselves in what looked to be a scene from *MASH*. It was like a war zone with people groaning on stretchers hooked up to IV drips, others leaning over vomiting into buckets, while some were lying on their backs writhing in agony as the doctors tended to their battered feet.

Max was seen to first as her feet were in a particularly bad way. She would need to have some of her peeling skin removed to prevent infection. She bravely let the doctors do what they had to do, wincing in pain. I didn't envy her but I wasn't feeling great myself and I became increasingly fatigued waiting my turn. The medical tent was so busy, there were no spare chairs or beds. All of a sudden, I felt so light-headed and weak, I couldn't stand up a moment longer. I collapsed to the ground and just wanted to curl up in a ball and sleep. I felt like my body was shutting down. At least I was in the right place to break down and the doctors immediately rushed to my aid and I heard Max crying out to ask if I was all right. I was carried onto a now available stretcher and given a rehydration drink but I threw it straight back up again.

'She needs an IV,' my hazed mind heard one of the doctor's say. Part of me thought, *No! I can't have the time penalty!* but I was so weak, I didn't even have the ability to muster the words to argue, all I wanted to do was sleep. There was a sharp prick as a needle was inserted into my arm and the IV drip began pumping saline solution into my body. Gradually I started to feel better and more human.

Max was allowed to leave the medical tent with her strapped-up feet but the doctors wanted me to rest for longer, eventually deciding I could return to my tent at 1 a.m.

'Are you sure you want to continue with the race?' one of them asked me before I left.

I didn't have to think twice, my answer was a resounding 'yes'. There was no way I was going to quit now.

I returned to my relieved campmates, who couldn't believe how much better I looked compared to when they had last seen me. I felt guilty telling Max and Louise that my health boost via the IV drip had cost us a 20-minute penalty, but they didn't mind in the slightest as they were just happy I was OK and able to continue. We had started as a team and wanted to finish as one.

I went to sleep that night feeling the best I had felt for days. We needed all the rest we could get as tomorrow was going to be the most challenging day of the race so far. The next stage was the 'Longest Day', the stage of the 52-miler. It really would be the longest of days, as it would take more than 24 hours to finish it; competitors are given two days for this stage. The cut-off time would be 40 hours, and it was up to competitors to decide if they would run the 52 miles all in one go, or break it up with a stop to sleep. However, there would be no campsite till you reached the end of the stage, so you would be sleeping under the stars with nothing but your sleeping bag for shelter from the sand-throwing wind. Our plan was to try to complete the distance in one go, as we would then have longer to rest at the next campsite before the fifth stage began, and would get better-quality sleep in the 'comfort' of the tent.

On the longest day, the start times were staggered, with slower runners setting off first and the faster elite runners at midday. We were set off in the first wave of runners and the early rise was a blessing in disguise as it meant we started before the heat of the sun really got going. It didn't take long for the faster runners to catch up with us and we were astounded by their pace as they overtook us. The lean, elite men made it look so easy as they swept past. They looked like they were floating across the sand doing a brisk three-mile run while we slogged on sinking into the terrain. Their backpacks also looked tiny, how had they managed to squeeze everything they needed into such a tiny bag when ours weighed 12 kg? In this leading pack was the indomitable Moroccan Lahcen Ahansal, who had won the race three times before and was the favourite to do it again. His younger brother, Mohamad, was his closest rival for the crown, which he had also won previously. The talented siblings grew up running round the Sahara so the MDS course was their native habitat. They were born to run through sand and heat, and we envied their effortless finesse. They would be at the next campsite with their feet up before we were even halfway there.

Thanks to the IV drip the day before, I was feeling much better. Now it was Max who was struggling, due to her sore, bleeding and blistered feet so we hung back to keep her company and support her as she winced in pain at every step. I couldn't help feeling sorry for Louise, who was feeling fine and continually held up by Max and me.

As the sun went down, we still had many miles to go so we pulled on our head torches to light our way. It was surreal running through the pitch black but the strong beams meant we could always see where we were treading. The only problem was remembering not to turn and look someone directly in the face when you spoke to them, as the beam of light from your torch could momentarily blind them. Seeing the other lights of the other runners bobbing along in front and behind us was an amazing sight, like fireflies doing a waltz. Above us the stars shone brightly and without the glare of any street lights, I could see constellation after beautiful constellation. It was a humbling, awe-inspiring sight. It felt much more pleasant to run through the night when the air was cooler so we decided to stick to our plan of running till morning. We'd just have a short rest at the next checkpoint, cook some food, and then keep running till we reached camp.

As we approached halfway, I was lagging behind the others, as the restoring effect of the IV drip had truly worn off and

I was back to feeling depleted and dejected, particularly as I hadn't been able to eat anything the night before. Max was also struggling but I was getting slower and slower, falling further behind her and Louise. Once again I felt utterly exhausted, every limb ached, even blinking was an immense effort. For the first time, a seed of doubt was sown in my mind and I thought, *I can't do this*. The more I thought it the more I believed it. Tears rolled down my face as I struggled to keep moving forward, I felt broken. Running any further felt physically impossible. I didn't have anything left. My fuel tank was completely empty, along with all the reserves. I wasn't going to make it to the next campsite and I certainly wasn't going to make it to the finish days later. I couldn't do it.

Max dropped back to find me hunched over dragging my feet along, using my poles for support. I voiced my doubts to her as I came to a stop and collapsed in the sand.

'I can't do this,' I groaned to her cradling my head in my hands as I sat on the soft ground. 'I can't go on, I can't run another step. I really don't think I can do this.'

Max turned to me but didn't give me sympathy or reassurance as I expected. She simply stated: 'Mimi, just think of all those people back at home who are expecting you to fail,' and then she walked off.

It sounds harsh but it was the best thing she could have said to me. Her words sunk in like pins popping the balloons of doubt in my mind. She was right – I couldn't fail. I couldn't go home and tell everyone that I wasn't good enough, that I had to quit because it was too hard. The *I can't* balloon burst, replaced by one floating to the fore of my mind, *I can*. I pulled myself together with a new sense of strength and determination, got myself back on my feet and continued with the girls to the next checkpoint. That was the first and last time I considered quitting. Now I was going to stay strong, no matter how painful it got; I was going to see this through to the end.

Finally arriving at our pit-stop at 9.45 p.m., the girls put me in my sleeping bag, boiled some water and made me a delicious cup of tea. Unfortunately I wasn't able to keep it down and proceeded to vomit over the poor guy who had the misfortune of sitting next to me. The medics came over to see me and were concerned about my condition, especially as I had just had an IV drip the day before. If they gave me another, I would have to be pulled from the race and that wasn't an option for me. Instead they gave me an anti-sickness pill and strongly suggested we rest there for the night instead of carrying on running without sleep as we had planned. Reluctantly, we agreed and looked for a spot to settle down for the night away from the strong winds. The best we could do was sleeping on the slope of a small sand dune. It didn't help much as we awoke six hours later covered in sand, layers of grains in our hair and stuck to our faces. It hadn't been a particularly relaxing experience, but I certainly felt better and a bit revitalised. We packed up and resumed our plod at 5.30 a.m., making good progress, but as the sun rose and it grew hot again, I began to think the wind that had battered us the night before wasn't so bad and wished it would return to cool us down.

Twenty-nine hours after we resumed running, we finally reached the end of the Longest Day, entering the campsite to cheers and rounds of applause from those who had already finished. This warm welcome made it all feel worthwhile and demonstrated the spirit of ultrarunners – everyone supports one another, no matter their pace; everyone is covering the same distance and battling the same demons to get to the end, regardless of how fast they manage to do it.

After surviving the Longest Day, I felt I had broken the back of the MDS. There was now 'only' a marathon and a half-marathon to go – that should be easy! The remainder of the route was also relatively flat so it wouldn't be as energy sapping as the earlier days. That's not to say it wasn't difficult: on the marathon day I felt constantly lethargic and dehydrated but our trio kept together, going at the pace Max could manage on her still afflicted feet. My frame of mind was completely different to the day before, now I was determined to finish regardless of the pain I was in.

Arriving at the penultimate checkpoint that day we encountered a man who was in a similar state to how I had been and suffering badly due to his trashed feet. The pain in his face was evidence enough of how sore they were. We stopped to check if he was OK as he was bent over being sick.

'I've had enough,' he said. 'I can't go on. I am going to pull out of the race.'

'You can't do that!' we told him. 'You have come this far; keep going to the campsite, as you might feel better after food and rest. Don't make a decision until tomorrow morning as you might feel better then and there will only be thirteen miles to go.'

'I can't do it,' he insisted. 'My feet are in agony, blister is covering blister, I have no skin left. Don't worry about me, ladies, you carry on.'

We reluctantly left him as the medical Jeep drove to his aid. We felt sad for him that he had managed to get so far and would have nothing to show for it if he quit. There were no medals for running 140 miles.

When we finally arrived at the camp, there was a jubilant atmosphere. Everyone was exhausted but they knew the worst was over. The following day, everyone would have six hours to cover 13 miles. Even if we had to walk the whole way, we would still have plenty of time to finish. We were beyond excited, we were set to join the ranks of the mighty endurance athletes who have completed the Marathon des Sables!

On the final day, there was a staggered start again, with the slowest set off at 8 a.m. and our turn at 9 a.m. Once again, the elite athletes stampeded past and we saw it was Lahcen who was going to take the victory again. You wouldn't have thought these athletes had been running mega-mileage for the previous five days, as they still looked fresh and full of energy. In comparison, Louise, Max and I were exhausted and limping. Despite the pain, our spirits were high, as we knew the finish would soon be in sight. We were given a further boost when a familiar voice sounded as a man bounded past us.

'Hello, ladies, remember me from yesterday? I didn't quit!' the man we had encountered the day before proudly declared as he raced by.

'Sorry, I can't stop,' he added. 'I was given some morphine and I have to keep running and get to the finish before it wears off!'

We were delighted he had carried on and it strengthened our own resolve to keep going.

With a mile and a half to go, we could finally see the finish line on the horizon.

'I think it's time we changed!' I told Max and Louise. 'We haven't carried those sparkly dresses all this way for nothing!'

We stopped to quickly pull on the disco diva outfits over our shorts to wear for the final mile. It was worth the effort to see the smiles it brought to the faces of our fellow weary runners as they saw us sparkling in the sun. Many must have thought they were hallucinating when they saw us looking as though we were a girl band on a shoot for a pop video, rather than Marathon des Sables finishers.

The final race village grew closer and we could see the giant hoarding of the finish and cheering crowds surrounding it.

The three of us held hands and ran across the line together as our glittery dresses shimmered and the crowd whooped and congratulated us. There aren't enough words to describe just how amazing that moment felt – marvellous, incredible, fantastic, life-affirming, euphoric – we'd done it!

Max was greeted by her husband, Russ, who had flown out to be at the finish and Louise by her friend Adrian. Meanwhile I was caught up in a huge hug by race director Patrick Bauer as he gave me a congratulatory kiss and hung my well-earned race medal around my neck. He was delighted at having pulled off another successful event and shared in our euphoria at finishing.

The carnival continued at a bar set up by the finish line and while the others clicked glasses of beers to toast our achievement, I could only stomach water while resting my head on the bar as I felt exhausted again. I wanted to share in the celebrations as I was so happy by what we had achieved but I felt overwhelmed with illness and felt similar to the day I had collapsed in the medical tent. I slept for the entire coach journey back to the hotel in Ouarzazate and once in our room, I collapsed on the bed still feeling awful. I went to use the loo – relishing the fact there was an actual toilet to sit on after a week of squatting in the sand to go – and was concerned when I noticed I was passing blood. I told Max I was worried and she urged me to go and see a doctor, as medics from the race were still available to consult at the hotel. Once again, I collapsed while waiting to be seen and had to be given another IV drip and a strong course of antibiotics. This time I was happy for the treatment. As the race was over, they could pump bag after bag into me, but they couldn't disqualify me or take away my medal now. Thanks to the medicine, I immediately started to feel better, apart from my aching muscles and sore feet.

That evening there was a prize-giving ceremony at the hotel held around the pool in the central courtyard. After applauding the leading athletes as they went up to receive their prizes, we decided to head back to our room to get ready for the rest of the evening's planned festivities to celebrate the end of the race. As I got out of the shower, I kept hearing the name 'Tuff Muthers' being called out from around the pool below our window. I paid no attention as I assumed I must be hearing things but then I heard it again: 'Would Tuff Muthers please come to the stage!'

'They're calling us!' I told Max, and we raced from our room pulling our clothes on as we went and grabbing Louise from her room on our way. Once at the courtyard we were amazed to be given the prize for the team with the best sense of humour. As far as I was concerned, that was better than coming first!

Once back at home, it was wonderful to be reunited with my family. My mother had done a great job looking after the kids and getting Ruaraidh back to health. She had struggled to keep the house as tidy as she knew I fastidiously liked it but that didn't matter – she had done her best and I was home. The children were excited to see me and were impressed with my medal, which they passed between them. However, they didn't seem remotely interested in the race or my experience, except to ask, 'Did you see a camel?' They were bursting to tell me what they had been up and I absolutely loved hearing all their news and to see Ruaraidh was on the mend. Tim was delighted when I called him on his fishing trip to tell him I had done it. He seemed relieved as if he was thinking, *Well, that's that. Mimi has achieved her goal and now she can hang up her trainers and return to being a full-time wife and mother*. But I felt I had been on a life-changing journey; how could I just go back to normal?

The following day, I had to do just that as I spent the entire morning catching up on the housework. As I sat recovering with a cup of coffee at the kitchen table, I couldn't believe what a difference a couple of days could make. This time last week, I had been an ultra-warrior, drinking my coffee outside a tent as the sun rose over the desert and about to embark on a gruelling run. Now I was back to being a housewife, looking at grey skies over the garden shed with just the ironing to tackle later. It almost felt as though the MDS had all been a dream. I had been on such an extraordinary adventure, but back at home, everyone else had carried on as before. Apart from Max and Louise, no one really understood what I had been through in the past week – the joyful highs, the painful lows and pushing my body past the brink of exhaustion. I still couldn't quite believe what I had achieved. I had completed the toughest footrace on earth, despite being ill and with the extra stress of my son being hospitalised in the build-up. If I could finish in those circumstances, what could I do when I was in top physical and mental health? It was a question I definitely wanted answered. It wasn't enough that I had done the MDS against the odds. I wanted to see what else I could achieve. The MDS hadn't got ultrarunning 'out of my system' as Tim had thought – it had ignited a passion for it. I wasn't going to give it up now. This was only the beginning.

CHAPTER FOUR

PROVING GOOD ENOUGH FOR BADWATER

Day eight continued: Warrington to Shrewsbury, 56 miles
After returning from the MDS a bona fide ultrarunner, I was still keen to do more, but I don't think Tim or I would ever have imagined it would one day lead me to attempt a Guinness World Record to run the length of Great Britain. Eight days into the JOGLE challenge, it was so far so good. But now there was a Karyn-shaped hole in the crew and there was some apprehension about who was coming to fill it – my husband. Alan, Becky and Phil had never met Tim before and I could tell they were wondering what he would be like and whether he would fit into the routine and rapport they had established. They had all been working so well together; Tim could come along and upset the whole dynamic.

I could tell they were feeling out of sorts when Alan made a map-reading mistake – the first of the entire journey.

We ended up running off-road across fields which slowed my progress and then the path became impassable as it was blocked with overhanging tree branches and dense undergrowth.

'Are you sure this is right?' I asked him. After double-checking the map to make sure we were heading in the right direction, we realised we had missed a turning that would have taken us on to a B road, rather than cross country. There was nothing for it but to turn around and head back the way we had come, the detour had cost us around half an hour. I was angry about it but I had to contain my rage rather than take it out on Alan, as it was an easy mistake to make. My mood also had something to do with Tim's imminent arrival. Running had always been 'my thing', separate from family life, so I was just as apprehensive as they were about how Tim would fit into the crew and whether he would upset the camaraderie that had been established. While I was extremely excited about seeing him, it would be weird having my husband crewing for me; I just wasn't used to him being part of that world.

It had been Karyn's idea for him to join us as she felt the crew wouldn't be able to manage with just the three of them after she left. Karyn and I had been friends for many years, so she knew Tim well and felt his background in the armed services and his map-reading skills would make him an asset to the crew, especially as he knew me inside out. Tim had also suggested he could be part of the crew when I was planning the world-record attempt, but I initially brushed off the idea as I wasn't sure. It wasn't that I didn't want him there or that I didn't want to spend time with him, it was just that running had become an opportunity for me to be something other than a wife and mother. Racing had given me back some of my identity which I had somehow lost after getting married and having children. When I ran I was Mimi – an ultrarunner, a competitor – not 'Mrs Anderson' or 'Emma/Ruaraidh/Harri's mum'.

It worried me that Tim might be too emotionally attached to be an objective member of crew. Would he be able to push me to keep going if I was really struggling and complaining that I couldn't go on? No one likes to see a loved one suffering and I wondered whether he would be able to urge me to get past the painful patches, or would he encourage me to stop to prevent me hurting myself further? Of course, you need your crew to stop you if you are gravely endangering your health but they need to be able to spot the difference between that, and when you're just having a dip that can be overcome. I wasn't sure if Tim would be able to make that judgement call when it was his wife in pain.

'You don't know what being a member of a crew involves or what running these kind of distances can do to me,' I said hoping to dissuade him. 'I don't know if you would enjoy it.'

'No – I don't know what it is like to crew because you never let me!' he replied. 'How can you expect me to support you when you never let me get involved?'

He was right and it was only then that I realised quite how much I had been shutting him out. I had wanted his help so I could train for my ultra-races but I had never let him share in my experiences. As he wasn't a runner, I had assumed he couldn't possibly understand what it took to be an indispensable crew member. I realised it was quite hurtful for me to push him away like that and to not have given him a chance.

'OK, let's give this a go,' I told him. 'But perhaps towards the middle of the run so I can get myself settled into a routine before you arrive.'

Having him join on day eight would let me start the challenge as normal – and it had the additional benefit of meaning we wouldn't be leaving Ruaraidh, now 20, home alone for too long. I feared left to his own devices, he could get up to no good! We didn't need to worry about our other two, as Emma had already moved out of home to start her own family and Harri was going to be on holiday in Spain with her best friend's family.

My thoughts were consumed with Tim's arrival as I ran towards Whitchurch and then suddenly, there he was. As the smaller of the two motorhomes overtook me to stop up ahead, I could see him hanging out the window waving at me enthusiastically. It was so wonderful to see him. I paused to give him a quick kiss before he drove on to meet me at my next planned rest stop. Seeing his face made all my worries about how he would cope go out the window. I just couldn't believe that he was here, everything was now perfect. I arrived to find him making spaghetti Bolognese in the motorhome as though he had been a member of the crew from day one. Stepping inside the vehicle and giving him a proper hug made me realise how much I had missed him. I could tell he was a little taken aback by my swollen appearance but he hid his concerns well to my relief, only commenting on my ankle which was still causing me to run with a slight limp.

'It looked like it was broken when I passed you running in the car,' he said.

'Nothing to worry about!' I reassured him. 'It's fine, just a little sore.'

The ankle was a long-standing niggle. Earlier in the year I had badly twisted it when taking part in a race in the Atacama Desert and I hadn't been able to run for weeks till it recovered. Ten weeks later I had taken part in a 100-mile race in South Africa where it flared up again, as it still wasn't strong enough. I kept going over on it so in the end I pulled out at 70 miles to avoid causing more damage to the ligaments and tendons. It was a tough call as I was the leading woman and in third place overall at the time, but my priority was JOGLE and I wanted, and needed it, to be recovered for that. So I wasn't surprised it was now causing me grief again and making my running style far from perfect, but I was able to keep moving at the desired pace and that was all that mattered.

Tim and I didn't have long to catch up, as the rest stop was a short one, giving me enough time to eat my lunch before heading out for the third four-hour stint of running that day. I was relieved to see Tim was getting on well with everyone and any apprehensive feelings in the group from the morning were banished. What a fool I had been to exclude him till now. In the years since I had first run the Marathon des Sables, I had taken part in races all over the world and become very much part of the running community, all without Tim by my side. It is something I now regret but I suppose it became a habit not to involve him in my running exploits, in the same way I rarely get involved in his fishing trips.

On returning from the MDS I was keen to take part in more ultra events but I could tell Tim was surprised and a little fed-up that it wasn't 'out of my system'. I knew it wouldn't be fair for me to expect him to carry on doing the bulk of the childcare at weekends to give me time to train for hours, so for the next two years, I carried on running but just went three or four times a week while he was at work and the children were at school or college. I entered two ultra-races to keep my toe in the water but chose ones in the UK so I wouldn't have to travel far away from home again.

In 2002, I ran the South Downs Trailwalker, a 62-mile (100-km) race over the South Downs in under 30 hours, and then in 2003, the Marathon of Britain, a 175-mile staged race over seven days from Warwickshire to Nottingham. At the Trailwalker, I ran as a team called Vintage 62 with Max, Rory Coleman and Paul Shields, the team name owing to the year we were all born. I felt good for most of the race, which was held on an extremely undulating off-road route across the South Downs from Queen Elizabeth Country Park in Hampshire to the finish at Brighton Racecourse. Imagine my delight when we finished as the fastest mixed team. I had never won anything based on my running performance before and it was completely unexpected. We had entered for the joy of taking part and never expected to be contenders for the prizes. It awakened a competitive spirit in me that I didn't know I had. I knew I was competitive with myself and what I could achieve, but I had never thought about my performance in relation to others before.

At the Marathon of Britain, I wondered if I might make a podium position again. This race offered a new challenge in that it was all self-navigated so it would test our map-reading skills to the extreme. Max and I planned to run together again, and for the first time, I began to become frustrated with our agreement of always running at the pace of the slowest runner, as she was going much slower than I would have liked. I could see other women bounding off ahead whom I was sure I could beat if only I was given the chance. As fate would have it, I would be, although I would rather the circumstances had been different. Three days into the race, Max was really struggling with severely blistered feet and I started to become increasingly concerned for her. Even in the MDS, I hadn't seen her look so bad. She then started suffering from sickness and stomach cramps and alarmed me by saying she was having hallucinations.

'I think I have taken too many pills,' she said clutching her stomach when she had to stop again. Unbeknown to me, she had been popping paracetamol and ibuprofen regularly to help her deal with her foot pain and she had lost track of just how many she had taken. Fearing she was close to an overdose and realising she was in no fit state to continue running, the race organisers decided it would be best if she were taken to hospital. I offered to go with her, but she urged me to finish the race for both of us.

I ploughed on and felt good, getting faster now I was running at my own pace. I started to pull back more and more weary competitors and used this to keep me pushing on. Instead of thinking of how far I had to go, I kept looking for the next female ahead of me and then focused on catching them up and overtaking. I didn't have any idea what position I moved up to, so I was delighted when I finished to be told I was the third-fastest female. There was a part of me that started to believe I might actually have a talent for running. I had been doing it because I loved the freedom and the exercise but now a more competitive streak was emerging.

If I kept training, what else could I achieve and how good could I be? They were questions I wouldn't be able to answer yet, as family life meant I couldn't commit to more training or major races that year. I did manage to fit in a marathon though, as luckily for me, my sister, Jacqui, and her husband lived in Rome, so I combined doing the Rome Marathon with a visit to see her and have a holiday with Tim. I finished in 3 hours and 34 minutes – a personal best (PB) I was proud of but it was tough as all my other races in the preceding years had been much longer distances. It felt like a sprint the whole way and I knew my heart lay in ultrarunning.

I craved my next challenge and, in 2004, it presented itself thanks to my friend Caroline Richards, whom I met when I moved to Kent. She was a keen mountaineer and had taken up running to improve her fitness, as she wanted to climb Mont Blanc. When she heard about a race – the Himalayan 100 – combining her two passions of mountains and running, she asked me if I wanted to go and run it with her. It is a staged 100-mile race over five days on the mountain roads near the border of Nepal. When she told me about it, it sounded too good an opportunity to miss. I had never been to that part of the world or run a mountain race at altitude. The event is described as a 'once-in-a-lifetime experience on the most spectacular running course in the world'. How could I resist? The scenic route passes through Sandakphu National Park and reaches 14,000 ft, providing amazing views of four of the five highest peaks in the world – Mount Everest, Kanchenjunga, Lhotse and

Makalu. Once again, I didn't think of how hard it would be, but just imagined myself running along the remote trails above the clouds surrounded by snowy mountain peaks. It would offer the chance to replicate the escapism and adventure I had experienced in the MDS, but in totally different conditions. Here, the challenge would not be the heat, but the gruelling inclines and descents and the thin air at altitude.

Running above sea level poses a number of challenges, because at high altitude there is less oxygen in the air. This means the lungs have to work harder to take in more oxygen and the heart has to put in more effort to pump it around the body. To acclimatise, the body produces more red blood cells to transport oxygen around the body. This is why many elite athletes train at altitude, as the additional red blood cells mean when they return to sea level, their body is more efficient at getting oxygen around the body. However, these changes don't occur overnight but after a prolonged period of training at altitude. We wouldn't gain these benefits from just five days running in the mountains. We would only have the pitfalls – finding it harder to breathe with our hearts beating faster the higher we climbed. As I have asthma, I was additionally concerned how this would affect my breathing, increasing the risk of me developing altitude sickness. But I was reassured by the fact this was an ultra-race with no cut-off times so there was no pressure to finish within a certain time each day. Everyone would be able to run at their own pace, even if that meant walking most of the way.

The decision made to run, I arranged for my mother to help Tim look after the children again while I was away. To my surprise, there was no resistance this time from Tim and no shock or disbelief over the fact I intended to run 100 miles in the mountains.

'This is total resignation,' he told me with a wry smile. 'I have now completely surrendered to your mad ultra-running plans.'

I swiftly got everything booked before he could change his mind and as I bought my plane ticket to Bagdogra, I felt a rush of nerves and excited anticipation that I hadn't felt since I entered the MDS. I had never travelled so far east before, let alone run through a world-famous range of mountains. In terms of the training, I was used to long-distance running by now so I didn't need to do much extra, although I did try to incorporate more hills to strengthen up my quads. The race would be broken up into five stages of 24, 20, 26, 13 and 17 miles – I knew I was well-capable of those distances, even though the mountainous terrain and lack of oxygen would make it harder.

Once I was there, the event exceeded all my expectations. The race starts at the foot of the mountains in the village of Manebhanjang, a small town with spectacular surroundings owing to its views of the giant peaks. It is a beautiful place but it was rather unsettlingly to be constantly confronted by armed guards due to its position on the Nepal–India border. Although far from being a tourist hotspot, it is a popular destination with mountain trekkers who often spend the night there before starting their journey. As you would expect of such a location in the great outdoors, facilities were few and far between so I had to join a huge queue for the only loo available at the bottom of the mountain before the race start. It was possibly the world's filthiest outside loo. Once I reached the front, I discovered the wooden cubicle was falling apart with a door that could barely close. Inside was a smelly squat loo with no toilet paper; instead there was a tap to wash yourself with. It wasn't at all what I was used to but I knew I had no choice but to get on with it, hold my nose and go as quickly as possible. I was thankful I had packed a hand sanitiser so I could clean my hands afterwards in an attempt to feel less filthy. It was another case of having to face the reality of just how unglamorous ultrarunning can be – but what was to come would make it worthwhile.

Once I'd escaped the loo, I joined Caroline and the other runners on the start line where a Tibetan blessing ceremony was held before we were given the signal to begin. Caroline and I had agreed in advance that we would run at our own paces rather than together so we were soon separated as we proceeded along a cobblestone path that started twisting, turning and undulating before becoming increasingly steeper. The scenery all around was breathtaking. We passed through Darjeeling tea plantations with the snowy peaks of the world's tallest mountains as our backdrop.

The higher we got the more laboured my breathing became and I had to start walking instead of running. It's not a race to do if you have a fear of heights, and going at a slower pace allowed me to take in my surroundings and see just how high I had climbed with the buildings in the village we had left behind becoming tiny dots below. There were terrifying drops off the side of some of the bends we took but the path was so wide, you never felt in any danger of going over the edge.

On the first day, I climbed up to 11,815 ft, covering 10,000 ft altitude gain, to reach the highest point in the race. It was a long and difficult climb to the top but completely worth the effort. When I reached the summit, the panoramic view that greeted me was so magnificent, it took my breath away. I felt as though I was on top of the world as my eyes feasted on the beauty below.

I dropped a short distance down to the first camp in Sandakphu, where I would be reunited with Caroline. A collection of rustic mountain huts would be our shelter for the night surrounded by more spectacular scenery. From the camp, you could see Everest, Lhotse, Makalu and Kanchenjunga, a sight to be savoured and enjoyed as we ate delicious local delicacies cooked and served to us by Sherpas. While the weather had been sunny and pleasant throughout the day, the temperature quickly dropped when darkness fell and the huts had no heating, so we wrapped up in as many clothes as we could wear before getting into our sleeping bags. Going to sleep that night there was so much for my brain to process, everything I had seen was so majestic and far removed from everything in my normal life. Hours later, I was jolted awake by the sound of one of the other girls sharing my hut screaming and turned to see her sat bolt upright in her bed. She woke the whole room up and when we all asked her what was the matter, she replied in terror: 'I felt something move across my face!'

None of us could go back to sleep after hearing that so we reached for our torches and shone them around the room to try to find the culprit. Finally the beams landed on a little mouse happily sitting on the window sill above her bed wondering what all the fuss was about, he then scuttled off leaving us in peace.

The following days continued to be magical and exhilarating with no two views ever the same. At times, you would be running along a plateau with rocky terrain all around; at others, running through lush, green pine forests alongside mountain springs. We would go through villages that seemed untouched by time with smoke pouring out of their chimney pots and the laid-back people going about their days. The locals always greeted us warmly as we passed through. They lived so cut off from the rest of the world, it wasn't often they welcomed tourists, or even saw people from outside the village. Women with beautiful, glossy black hair would sit crossed-legged by the roadside, breaking up rocks to be used to fill potholes in the road surface we ran on, while their excited children bounded over to run with us for a few metres as we weaved through the cobbled streets.

The whole thing was amazing but also one of the toughest races I have ever done thanks to the altitude. At times, my breathing was so laboured it felt like I was running with a sock in my mouth; I simply couldn't get enough oxygen into my lungs. I was glad there was no pressure to reach each stage in a certain time, as this allowed me to walk if I needed to, giving me more time to take in my surroundings and chat to my fellow competitors. Strangers quickly become friends when you're hiking and camping together in a place cut-off from civilisation, where you are all striving to cover 100 tough miles. With a love of running in common, chatting about the sport breaks the ice, and then as you travel together you end up talking about anything and everything. The kind of bonds that are quickly formed during such events is another reason why I love ultrarunning; it has enabled me to make many friends around the world.

As more men than women competed in ultras at this time (although the balance is slowly shifting now, which is great news) and Caroline and I weren't running together, I would inevitably spend much of my time in male company. This would lead some people back home – often the partners of friends – to say things like 'I wouldn't let my wife go off gallivanting around the world sharing a tent with strange men', implying these trips were akin to a debauched Club 18–30 holiday. Tim trusted me and he knew when I went away I would always be focused on the race. Besides, we were happily married so there was never a thought given to a naughty liaison with another competitor, and even if there had been, an ultra event would be the last place I would want to indulge in one. By the time I hit the sack at night, all I wanted to do was sleep; I wouldn't have had the time, energy or inclination for anything else!

Just as during the MDS, for the entire race in the Himalayas I didn't have any means of contacting Tim and this made me miss him more and realise how much I loved him. In the modern era of mobile phones and text messaging, I'm not sure many couples get to experience how 'absence makes the heart grow fonder' in this way any more.

While I loved my time in the mountains, by the final day, I was looking forward to finishing and returning to my family. The last stage is a continual descent to finish in the picturesque village of Mirik, which lies on the banks of a beautiful lake with the mountains towering above and temples and monasteries set on the hillsides. As I hadn't been competitive during the race, I was thrilled to finish third-fastest female. That was the icing on the cake of what had been a truly fantastic race experience, shared with my friend Caroline.

During my time at the Himalayan 100, the name of another race kept cropping up among my fellow runners – the Badwater Ultramarathon. It was a badge of honour for the few who had completed it and I made a note to myself to find out more about this revered race when I returned home. I discovered it was the stuff of ultrarunning legend, 'a true challenge of the champions', the pinnacle of long-distance running. First held in America in 1987 with a handful of runners, it had grown to become globally famous, attracting hundreds who wanted to see if they had what it takes to conquer it. It begins 282 ft below sea level in the Badwater Basin in Death Valley, California, the lowest point in the western hemisphere, before going through three mountain ranges to finish 135 miles later in the portals of Mount Witney, 8,300 feet above sea level (the original route had been 146 miles to climb to the summit of Mount Whitney, 14,505 ft above sea level, the highest point in the contiguous United States, but snow and ice often made the mountain paths impassable so the route was amended to avoid the race being cancelled in the event of adverse weather). As if the epic distance and the extremely hilly terrain weren't enough to make this one of the toughest races on the planet, also thrown into the mix is unbearably hot weather, comparable to running in a hot oven. Temperatures in the desert valley can soar to 54°C, and the race is purposefully staged in July to ensure a maximum chance of a heatwave. Competitors run on long, tarmac highways with no shade and the sunrays reflecting off the tarmac to increase the heat even more. Badwater legend has it that trainers can melt on the roads because the tarmac is so burning hot. Some of the best ultrarunners in the world have been defeated by the gruelling course and boiling conditions. Oh, and did I mention you have to do it all non-stop? Brief rests are allowed but there's no time to sleep and no overnight camping.

If ultrarunning was an Olympic sport, coming first at Badwater would be like winning the gold medal. When I looked up the names of those who had won it up until 2004, it was a who's who of ultrarunning icons – Marshall Ulrich, Dean Karnazes, Pam Reed. All these champions had not just conquered the course and the conditions, but beaten fellow competitors who were the cream of the ultrarunning crop, as not just anyone can run at Badwater. You have to earn your right to race by meeting the strict qualification standards or, if you're lucky enough, be invited to take part having previously proved your mettle as an ultrarunner, Ironman or extreme adventurer. So only the best endurance athletes in the world make it to the start. If they then manage to finish in under 48 hours, they win the coveted Badwater Buckle, one of the greatest prizes in the world of ultrarunning.

Of course, learning all this completely whet my competitive appetite. I wanted to earn the right to take part and I wanted that buckle. The race itself sounded brutal and demanding but that only increased my desire to do it.

It would be another test of what I could do when the heat was – quite literally – on.

However, as I had only taken up ultrarunning three years before, my achievements so far weren't nearly enough to impress the Badwater organisers. I would have to prove myself as a contender in order to gain a place in the 2005 race. How was I going to do that? After chatting to ultrarunning friends, I was told the Grand Union Canal Race (GUCR) was deemed a tough enough qualifying race for Badwater. If I could finish the 145-mile race, running non-stop from Birmingham to Little Venice in central London, in under 40 hours, I would be able to apply. The gauntlet was laid down; it was time to start training. Given the route was entirely flat along the canal and would be held on a British May bank holiday – meaning it would be much more likely to rain than be hot and sunny – some might say it was an easy option as a Badwater qualifier. But then those people are unlikely to have ever tried running 145 miles in less than 40 hours before. It would be tough. In fact, ultrarunning on a flat route can be more difficult than a hilly one as steep inclines can offer a bit of respite from running, as often you have no choice but to walk up them. In comparison, when running along a flat towpath there are no excuses to walk, putting much more pressure on the hips and legs, especially over 145 miles. To add to the difficulty at the GUCR, competitors aren't allowed to stop and rest for more than 40 minutes at a time, otherwise they would be disqualified, and crew aren't allowed to run with them until they reach Navigation Bridge in Milton Keynes, nearly halfway at 70.5 miles. This checkpoint must also be reached within 19 hours to avoid disqualification, as all competitors must finish within 45 hours.

It was a daunting prospect for me. I had run 156 miles at the MDS and 175 at the Marathon of Britain, but these had both been broken up into stages with overnight stops in between. In the GUCR, I would have to cover 145 miles with barely any chance to rest and the added pressure of running against the clock. Most people who had run it before told me it would be near impossible to get under 40 hours on my first attempt. Many experienced runners often failed to complete the race, let alone do it in the Badwater qualifying time. But you should know by now how much I love to prove people wrong, especially when they say something is impossible. I always think beyond impossible. What's the point in setting limits on what you can do before you have even tried to do it? I was going to give it my best shot, with the chance to run the Badwater Ultramarathon as my prize.

Or, as Tim put it, once again astounded by my intentions: 'You want to do a challenging and painful long-distance race, in order to qualify to do an even more challenging and painful long-distance race?'

I trained hard for months and found it much easier to fit the runs in now our children were aged 19, 17 and 11 so were no longer as reliant on Tim and me. Access to the internet had improved so I joined various online running forums to try to glean training and recovery tips, as I wanted to be as physically and mentally prepared as possible. Max and Andy Rivett (who holds the male world record for the fastest time running Land's End to John o'Groats) agreed to crew for me, which was fantastic. By the time the May Bank Holiday came around, I was feeling fit and confident. I had done all I could to prepare and I felt capable of finishing in time to earn a place at Badwater.

The night before the start, I was relaxed as I had a meal with Max and Andy at our hotel in central Birmingham, which was a two-minute walk from the race start. I felt so relaxed I decided to do something I have never done on the eve of an ultra before – have a glass of wine. One glass led to another as the three of us were having such a good time chatting and laughing; before I knew it, I must have had close to a bottle and was completely drunk. At the time I thought it was hilarious that I might have to start the race tipsy and staggered off to bed feeling amused with myself. Reality hit with a headache when I woke up early the next morning after four hours' sleep, still with my make-up on from the night, as I hadn't removed it before crashing out in my inebriated state. I was still feeling tipsy but now that was no longer amusing, it was mortifying.

'What was I thinking?' I berated myself. I could have jeopardised everything I had been training for, not to mention a place at Badwater. I felt totally ashamed. How could I have been so stupid? My parents were going to be at the start to see me off and I couldn't let them know what a drunken fool I had been. I scrubbed my teeth repeatedly before I left and hoped they wouldn't be able to smell any alcohol on my breath, or notice that I was still a little giddy.

There was also the fear that once the effects of the alcohol had worn off, I would start to feel hung-over, and the last thing anyone wants to do with a hangover is run 145 miles. As well as my water, I also packed my bum bag with extra energy gels, so I could at least try to rehydrate and keep topped up on salt and carbs. The instructions said they could be taken every 45 minutes, something I wouldn't normally find necessary, but on this occasion, I was going to take them every three-quarters of an hour like clockwork.

As if to rub my face in my mistake even more, the race registration was held in a pub – the Red Lion, near the start on the Gas Street Basin. Luckily I had registered the night before and been given my number and race T-shirt, so I could go straight to the start line and attempt to look normal rather than go inside and see and smell more alcohol. As my parents came over to see me, I was relieved when they didn't seem to notice the smell of wine on me when they gave me a good luck hug. With their best wishes ringing in my ears, I started to feel confident again. Maybe it was because I was still drunk, but I felt invincible and ready to run.

Having never run when under the influence of alcohol before, it was strange to be feeling tipsy when the race began at 6 a.m. I was still angry with myself for allowing this to happen and worried I had screwed up all my race plans. But as the opening miles went by, it didn't seem to be adversely affecting me; so far, my feet seemed to be flying as the miles went by. I couldn't change what had happened so now I had to focus on the task at hand – keep moving and keep taking on the gels and water to stave off any energy slumps as I sobered up.

There was a good atmosphere among the other runners and I enjoyed the route as we passed colourful narrowboats along the canal and waved to people on board as they navigated locks. Occasionally, there was a little steeplechasing to be done as we dodged fishermen sat out by the water with their long poles stretching back across the path. It was all very pleasant and serene with the canal banks surrounded by blossoming spring flowers and ducks swimming along the water trailed by their ducklings.

Luckily, my body seemed to be coping, despite my liberal wine-intake the night before, and I was making good progress. It was an easy course to navigate since it is along the canal but I had to have my wits about me and carry a map of the course because at various points it was necessary to cross a bridge and run on the other side of the canal. On numerous occasions, I saw runners across the water who had missed bridge crossings and had to turn back after realising their mistake, adding extra miles to their journeys which their tired legs could well do without.

I reached Navigation Bridge well within the cut-off time and it was wonderful to meet up with my crew again. They didn't need to run with me yet, as I was running with Rob Cousins, another competitor who I had met along the course. As we were going at the same pace, it made sense to stick together so we could keep one another company during the long, lonely stretches between checkpoints.

As darkness fell and Rob and I continued to run through the night, our head torches lighting the way, my 'witching hour' began around 2 a.m. This was when I had to work my hardest to stay awake. My crew anticipated my fatigue and gave me a strong coffee at every checkpoint to help me fight off the sleep demons. Despite the caffeine, by 4 a.m. I was really struggling and my body just wanted to shut down and go to sleep. I tried to focus on the sound of my and Rob's footsteps as I desperately tried to keep my eyes open. Suddenly I was wide awake when the rhythm of our footsteps changed and Rob surged ahead. He was running with his arms wide open like an aeroplane, flying down the canal as though he intended to take off by leaping across the water. There was a moment of panic as I chased after him and grabbed his arm to stop him jumping into the canal. He looked so bewildered as he came out of his trance – his fatigue had caused him to hallucinate. Although we were able to laugh later at his belief he could fly, at the time it was pretty scary. Thankfully I managed to get him safely to the next checkpoint where we had a 20-minute break with our crews before continuing. We both felt much better after the short break for food, and my crew helped me change into warmer and drier clothing as efficiently as a Formula One team dealing with a race car at a pit-stop.

Running with their support and Rob's company made such a difference and helped the miles pass by much more quickly and I started running faster than I had in the first half, putting me on track for the holy grail of distance racing – a negative split.

The sun came back up and we ran into a new day. We passed through Kings Langley onto Watford; knowing I was now within the M25 gave me a big boost. Central London didn't feel that far now – only a mere 32 miles to go!

As we got closer to the centre of the capital, the towpaths that had been tranquil and devoid of people for much of the way started to get busier with cyclists and dog walkers and others just out for a Sunday jog or stroll. As I could see the London skyscrapers on the skyline getting closer, I could smell the finish line. I knew it couldn't be far now and then finally I saw the blessed banner 'FINISH' strung across the path in Little Venice close to London Zoo.

It was just after 9 p.m. when I was finally able to stop. I was the second woman across the line and one of only 23 finishers out of the 54 runners who had started. But what of my time, which was all that mattered to me? Had I qualified for Badwater? I didn't need to check my own watch, as people started congratulating me as soon as I crossed the line. I had done it. Both Rob and I had finished in 39 hours and 39 minutes. Now I could apply to take part in Badwater, my dream race. Max gave me a congratulatory hug and I thanked her for helping me. She had been a fantastic crew member and friend.

'It's amazing considering how you felt when you started. Perhaps you should get drunk before a race more often!' she joked. But I had learned my lesson in that respect, from now on: it would be sparkling water only before a big race!

My application for Badwater was posted in January 2005 and I had an agonising six-week wait to find out if it had been accepted based on my Grand Union time. I was elated when a letter arrived inviting me to take part. I had to pinch myself; it was like finding the golden ticket to visit Willy Wonka's Chocolate Factory. I was going to be part of something big and exclusive – but I mustn't forget challenging and painful. The pre-race pack did not sugar-coat what was in store. It stated just how dangerous the event could be, due to the health risks of running in the extreme heat:

This 135-mile race is the most physically taxing competitive event in the world. It also has considerable medical risks. All runners and crews must appreciate these two facts both before and during the race. Heat illness and heat stroke are serious risks. These can cause death, renal shut-down and brain damage. It is important that runners and crews be aware of the symptoms of impending heat illness.

If the heat didn't get you, there was also the danger of altitude sickness when you're scaling the mountains. The race information warned: 'The high altitude plus exertion can produce various degrees of altitude sickness. This can lead to severe lung and brain swelling, and even death. The main treatment is rest, and especially to get to a lower altitude.'

There was also a warning on preparing your feet to be able to run on pavements that could reach temperatures of 93°C, as 'blisters are also a problem on this course'. Blisters sounded like the least of my worries, as the booklet ended with the not-so-reassuring final paragraph: 'There are no aid stations. Know where your limits are and know your body. Your acceptance of invitation to this race declares that you are aware of the risks and potential health problems.'

It wasn't easy reading but it didn't put me off. Previous runners over the years had proved it could be done and there hasn't been a fatality in the race's history. I made it my aim to finish in less than 48 hours so I could win the Badwater Buckle. I didn't want to go through it all and come away empty-handed.

I knew from doing the MDS that I could run in high temperatures, and I had managed it when I had been unwell. However, the Death Valley highways would be even hotter than the Sahara and I wouldn't be able to get an IV drip in order to continue like I had at the MDS if I became severely dehydrated. Having a drip at Badwater equalled instant disqualification. It was vital that I acclimatised my body to running in such extreme heat in the months prior to the race.

There were a few British people who had completed the race in previous years who I was able to turn to in order to find out how they prepared. Thank heavens for the internet, as I was also able to join forums to chat to former competitors from around the world to see what they recommended. Training in the desert was a common tip, but living in Kent, not a great option for me and I couldn't afford to go abroad for warm-weather training as Badwater was already going to be an expensive trip. But all was not lost, as I was told one of the main ways people acclimatised was by spending time in a sauna – some even ran on treadmills inside them. So the sauna at my local gym became my second home and my sessions there in the month before the race would be anything between 30 minutes to two hours. There was no way I could get a treadmill inside so instead I did some stretching and sits-ups to pass the time. When the heat became too intense, I would nip outside for a few minutes to cool down.

Alongside my training, I had to arrange my travel plans and organise a crew to support me. It is compulsory for each runner to have at least two crew members with a vehicle to help them along the 135-mile route, so I asked Karyn and Tim Welch if they would be willing to come and help me. Both know me extremely well and, as Tim was an experienced ultrarunner himself, he knew what it would take to help me finish.

They would meet me every mile to spray me down with water, replenish my fluids and feed me, keeping a constant check on my health to ensure I wasn't in danger of overheating. They had to be clued up on the signs and symptoms of heat exhaustion and altitude sickness. They would not be allowed to trail me in the support vehicle but always had to 'leapfrog' my position to stay one step ahead. They were permitted to run but not cycle – alongside me from the first checkpoint in Furnace Creek at 17.2 miles, but they couldn't offer any other assistance. For example, it was forbidden for them to hold a parasol over my head to provide any shade from the sun, or physically support me if my legs started to wobble – there could be no Alistair Brownlee-style heroics here, carrying someone across the line if they faltered in the final metres. The race organisers are very insistent that while competitors need crew for their health and safety, they still have to complete the entire race on their own two feet, without 'any type of physical assistance'.

Leaving Tim behind once again to man the home front, I flew to Las Vegas in July 2005 with Karyn and Tim W. to face my ultimate battle. On the flight, we were surrounded by holidaymakers, including quite a lot of stag and hen parties. When the latter groups landed, they headed off to get stocked up on booze, but our priority was water. At the airport, we picked up the four-by-four we had hired as my support vehicle and then went straight to the supermarket to fill the boot with food and 150 litres of water. The following morning, we drove to Furnace Creek visitors' centre for registration and a pre-race meeting, where I would meet my fellow competitors and be given a full safety briefing. When we arrived, the whole place was buzzing with anticipation. There were 81 athletes in total due to take part and it was inspiring to hear some of their stories of how and why they had qualified. Some were seasoned ultrarunners who had done Badwater before and were back for more, others were attempting it for the second time after a dreaded DNF (Did Not Finish) in a previous year. Many were Badwater virgins like me (or rookies, as the Americans called us), drawn to the challenge of running in such an extreme environment.

The international field of athletes included 14 women and 67 men and there were countless inspiring stories of what they had achieved and overcome to be there. Two competitors were blind and would be running with guides; another was taking part after suffering a fractured back in a car accident just three years before; others were former members of the Armed Forces who had been in combat.

One was an amputee who had lost a leg on a landmine in the Vietnam War.

The oldest runner was a fellow Brit, grandfather Jack Denness, who was a remarkable 70 years of age. I hadn't met him before but I had heard of him as he was also from Kent. He had taken part 11 times before and wasn't going to let his age stop him joining in again this year. Meanwhile, the youngest participants were Americans Judit Pallos, 28, and Scott Jurek, 31. Now world-renowned for his running feats, Scott was a rising star in the ultra world at that time as he had won the Western States 100 – a famous ultra in the USA – seven years in a row despite his young age. Great things were expected of him in his first attempt at Badwater – although I don't think anyone quite expected him to excel as much as he did. He ended up not just winning the race, but smashing the previous course record by more than 30 minutes in the process with his time of 24 hours 36 minutes.

Looking around the room at the pre-race briefing, it was awe-inspiring to be in the company of so many people who had such grit, determination and endurance. I was also star-struck to see so many former Badwater champions, who were now my peers. There was Marshall Ulrich, a renowned mountaineer and adventurer who had won it on four previous occasions, and Pam Reed, who had not only set an amazing female course record of 27 hours 56 minutes and 47 seconds in 2002, but had won the whole race outright.

She repeated this winning feat in 2003 leaving all male and female competitors trailing in her wake.

I lapped up the stories from the runners and crew members who had done it before, hearing their highs and lows and trying to snatch any last-minute tips. Then all the runners were brought together on stage to a round of applause, followed by one of the Badwater rituals – having our 'mugshots' taken holding our race numbers. I was trembling with excitement and beaming with pride as I posed for my snap. I couldn't believe I was joining the ranks of ultrarunning legends – now I just had to prove myself worthy of my place by finishing the race. We were each asked by a reporter to sum up how we were feeling ahead of the event and there was just one word that sprang to mind for me, 'marvellous'.

Each competitor's start time depended on their qualifying time, and runners would be set off in three waves at 6 a.m., 8 a.m. and 10 a.m. I was shocked to have been put on the 10 a.m. start with all the top runners including Jurek, Reed and Ulrich. It was an honour but also a terrifying prospect; I was not in their league.

The next morning, as I stood on the start line decked out in white racing kit with my legionnaire hat on to protect me from the sun, I still couldn't believe I was about to be set off with the world's best ultrarunners. Surely there had been some mistake? I wasn't good enough to toe the line with the likes of them.

It was interesting to observe the different race preps of these elite athletes. Some were 'in the zone', seemingly blocking out all around them and only focusing on the road ahead. Others were more relaxed and chatty, smiling at the surrounding supporters there to see them off. I hovered at the back of the group, a mixture of nerves and excitement. After all the training and the hard work to get here, this was it, race time.

Both the Canadian and American national anthems were enthusiastically sung followed by a ten-second countdown and then we were off. The elite runners seemed to shoot off like bullets and I had to remind myself not to panic and to just focus on running at my own pace. I wasn't used to being at the very back of the pack in the opening miles of a race, but I had to keep reminding myself this was no ordinary race and it was no shame to be last when the runners ahead were all ultra gods and goddesses.

The temperature was already rising as we rounded the base of the Amargosa mountain range. The runners on the earlier starts had the fortune of running this section in the shade, but now the sun had risen over the peak and beat down on us relentlessly. It didn't feel like too long before I started catching up with some of the slower 8 a.m. runners and that gave me a mental boost. I tried to focus on pulling back the runners ahead rather than on the long, seemingly never-ending stretches of road to be travelled. I didn't think about the total distance I had to run, but just focused on making it to each checkpoint. Breaking the race down into each stage made it seem a lot more manageable.

It wasn't the distance that fazed me but the heat. It was so unbearably hot, hotter than I had experienced at the MDS and even the sauna training hadn't prepared me for it. By the time I reached the first checkpoint at Furnace Creek Ranch, just over 17 miles into the race, the temperature had already risen to a sweltering 48°C. The relatively flat section to the next mountain range was completely exposed to the relentless sun beams. My crew continued to meet me every mile to change my drinks, give me electrolyte pills and spray me with water to cool me down – but as it got even hotter it seemed to evaporate before it even hit my face.

At the 30-mile point, the hills I had heard so much about in the build-up began. I ran up and up and up, zigzagging round and round hairpin turns cut into the rock face with the top never seeming to be getting any closer. I'd have loved to have had some walking poles to aid my upward motion but they weren't allowed. Looking down at my legs as I trudged on, I noticed my skin had broken out in large, blotchy red patches.

'You got hives,' a member of a fellow competitor's crew told me in an American drawl as they overtook me when I paused for a drink. 'Happens all the time at Badwater.'

Luckily for me, Tim had come prepared with lightweight sun-protective trousers, so I pulled these on to shield my skin as the climb continued up and up till I reached

4,965 ft above sea level. This was followed by a nine-mile section that took me back down 1,640 ft. I had expected the downhill to offer some respite but it was just as tough as the uphill. My hamstrings felt under strain and it was a battle to stay in control as the road twisted and turned downwards and gravity pulled me at a faster pace than I felt safe or comfortable doing.

To make things even more tricky, it was now dark. Unfortunately, this didn't result in much of a drop in the temperature – it was still close to 30°C. I had to concentrate on where I was going but I couldn't resist stealing glances at the view up ahead. The lights of the faster competitors and their support vehicles were snaking up the next hill ahead of me, creating a mesmerising, beautiful and bright cavalcade.

Tim and Karyn started to take it in turns to run with me and we were lit up like Christmas trees so passing cars could spot us from a long way off. I was so glad of Karyn's constant chatter as it distracted me from the aches and pains and the distance still left to run. True to form, she'd talked non-stop to everyone she had encountered so far and told me all about the other runners and crew members she had met. I didn't have the energy to join in much of a conversation but I enjoyed hearing her speak. As I listened, I looked overhead at a beautiful blanket of stars and occasionally spotted a shooting star streaking across the sky. Each time, I tried to point them out to Karyn but she kept missing them, as she was too busy chatting.

We reached the Panamint Valley and the road continued up and up, leaving the valley far below us as we twisted and turned on more sharp switchbacks. A perk of running through the night was that we then had the pleasure of witnessing the sun rise. A new day was dawning and I was excited to see what it would bring. Of course, it brought heat, lots of it, and my energy levels dipped the higher the mercury rose. My quads burned and I had three large blisters aggravating my feet. I felt so tired after running through the night but I was determined not to complain to Karyn and Tim. This was what I had signed up for and what endurance running was all about. They were brilliant at encouraging me and tending to my blisters and giving my aching muscles a quick rub at rest stops. To combat my fatigue, Karyn suggested I have a can of Red Bull. It tasted disgusting but the caffeine was just what I needed for a second wind.

After 100 miles, the route began to flatten out again but it didn't feel much better for my body or mind. Painful though they were, at least the ups and downs of the hills had provided some variation, as well as stunning views. Now a straight road towards Lone Pine stretched off into the horizon, flanked by the mountains and salt flats glistening in the sun, which continued to burn down from high overhead. The road seemed to be never-ending; at times, it felt like I was running on the spot as the surroundings didn't change and the end never seemed to get any closer. Luckily music was to be my salvation: listening to tunes on my mp3 player took my mind off it. Finally I reached a right turn towards the penultimate checkpoint at the Dow Villa Motel and then progressed to the Whitney Portal Road at mile 122. I was relieved there was now only a half-marathon to go – but the organisers had kindly saved the steepest hills till last. The road to the finish line started at 3,610 ft and finished at 8,360 ft. While the elite runners had passed this section hours earlier in daylight, for me it was dark again. But I actually found this useful, as it meant I couldn't see quite how steep the hill was. I was so, so tired after nearly 40 hours of being on my feet with no sleep, my pace started getting slower and slower and I had to keep dragging one foot in front of the other. I was struggling to keep my eyes open so much, I was practically sleepwalking. The sleep deprivation and darkness meant my mind started playing tricks on me and I started hallucinating.

'Look at that giant teddy bear,' I would mumble to Karyn, when we were in fact passing a large rock or tree. I sounded as though I was drunk.

'How about a Pro Plus?' she asked, handing me a caffeine tablet. It was just what I needed to perk me up.

Karyn and Tim had been taking it in turns to stagger up the hill with me while the other went ahead in the four-by-four. With one mile to go, they parked the car so they could both join me for the final effort. We eventually turned a bend to see the glorious 'FINISH' sign nestled among the pine trees. Spectators, including those who had already finished and their crews lined the home straight to cheer me on and tape was held up for me to break as I crossed the finish line – a wonderful touch not just reserved for the champions.

I checked the clock. My finishing time was 41 hours and 5 minutes – the Badwater Buckle was mine! I was exhausted but elated. I had finished 23rd out of the 81 starters, was the sixth-fastest female and the first Brit. Sixty-seven others finished within the 60-hour cut-off time, an 83 per cent finishing rate, which I was told was especially impressive, as that year the conditions had been 'particularly challenging, even for this event and its hostile venue'. The highest official temperature when we had been running was 47.8°C on the first day. I couldn't have been prouder to be one of the finishers and to be part of a race in which history was made as Scott Jurek set a new course record.

Gaining the Buckle was like receiving an Olympic gold medal or world record for me. I was proud and honoured to have earned my place running with the best endurance athletes in the world – not bad for a housewife who had only been running for the past five years.

CHAPTER FIVE

WINNING AND LOSING IN THE ARCTIC

Day nine: Shrewsbury to Hereford, 62 miles

Day nine into JOGLE and the wheels were starting to come off. Not just metaphorically for me, but also for the bikes the crew were using. The pedals had been pounded for so many miles, the machines were starting to fall to pieces. The brakes had gone on one and the chain had snapped on another. Tim was forced to spend the last section of the day pushing his now useless bike beside me, which wasn't very comfortable for him.

In contrast, I was feeling fantastic. It was a beautiful, clear evening where I had witnessed a glorious sunset as I ran into the night and I was happy to keep pushing on. So imagine my frustration when I saw the motorhomes parked up ready and waiting for me a few miles earlier than planned. I wasn't a happy bunny, as it would mean stopping when I was feeling good, and then having to run the extra miles in the morning when I was tired. I was seriously miffed as I came to a halt but I had to go with what the crew thought best, as they had identified this as the best spot in the area to park for the night. The more tired I was getting the more I had to make an effort not to be grumpy with my dedicated crew. I tried to look on the positive side – at least stopping now meant I would get to sleep earlier. Ironically, we had parked up outside a bike shop but our late arrival and early departure meant the store wouldn't be open while we were there. Becky joked we could break-in to steal the parts we needed to mend the bikes.

'Well, I'll leave you to it; I need to sleep!' I told them and crashed out for a few precious hours.

Day ten: Hereford to Congresbury, 61 miles

The following morning I was exhausted and I set off in the early hours still feeling annoyed about having to cover the extra miles I could have easily done the night before. The crew had decided it would be quicker to buy new bikes rather than waste time buying parts and repairing the old ones, so they split up. Alan and Tim would visit a bike shop and catch up with us later. The staff must have thought they were on the run from the law, such was their urgency to buy them and get on their way again.

'We'll take this one!' they shouted of the first one they saw after rushing in as soon as the store opened. 'No, we can't come back and get it tomorrow! We need it now!'

We were all starting to feel the pressure of the ticking clock on the world record. Every unplanned delay was eating into the time we had meticulously scheduled to stay on track. But if I thought the hiccups we'd had so far had been stressful – from cystitis-induced toilet breaks to roadwork enforced detours and broken down bicycles – then things were about to go from bad to worse.

The day had started out so promisingly, the crew were back on their bikes and I had survived the first four-hour run of the day, which I always found the hardest, as my body was still warming up and I knew I had a whole day of running ahead of me. It had helped that I had crossed the border into Wales – the third country to run through during the challenge. Conditions were ideal as I ran through the scenic Wye Valley surrounded by fields of sheep and running under arches of trees that intertwined over the path above me. I was starting to feel positive again and was enjoying my pretty surroundings.

At my lunch stop I was treated to a visit by my two sponsors – Tom Atwood and Andrew Ross from ICG and Cazenove Capital respectively – who had generously sponsored my challenge. Each company had given £5,000, which had paid for the hire of the motorhomes, food, petrol and other essential kit. After chatting to them while I ate my lunch, I ran on alone along a section of road towards Chepstow while the rest of the crew packed up and bid Tom and Andrew farewell.

There was no pavement and little traffic as I ran but I hugged the roadside as much as possible to be safe and was decked out as usual in my high-vis clothing. Before Becky had caught me up on the bike, a black car suddenly sped towards me out of nowhere and before I could react – *BAM!* – I heard a smash and felt a surge of pain in my right arm. The passing car had struck me with such force, its wing mirror broke off and I saw it smash on the road ahead of me. I was forced to stop in shock and pain but the driver didn't hesitate. They drove off without stopping to check if I was harmed. I was the victim of a hit-and-run. I couldn't believe this criminal behaviour. How could a driver be so reckless? I wish I had seen the licence plate to report them to the police but it had all happened so quickly I hadn't noticed. I couldn't even recall what make of vehicle it was, only the colour.

At that moment, I was more concerned about my arm and whether or not it was broken. If it was, my world record attempt was over. Becky rushed over to help me as I nursed my bruised and swollen arm at the side of the road, cursing the driver who had done this to me. When the rest of the crew caught up, they couldn't believe it when I told them I had been hit by a car and that the driver hadn't even stopped.

'Surely they must have heard the bang on impact and noticed the loss of their wing mirror?' Phil said, spotting the smashed part on the concrete.

Tim was particularly upset and angry. As my husband, he felt he had failed to protect me – although of course there is nothing he could have done. He had to take himself away for a few moments to compose himself as he didn't want me to see him when he was so emotional, in case it made me feel worse. Becky looked over my bruised and battered arm and reached for the first-aid kit, although there was little within it that could really help me. There was no blood and I could still move my fingers so I didn't think it was broken.

'Do you think we should go to the hospital just to be sure?' she asked me.

'We don't have time for that!' I said.

It could take hours to get an X-ray once we got to an A & E and it was unlikely a doctor would be willing to patch me up and send me on my way when I told them I was planning to run another few hundred miles nursing such an injury. If we went to a hospital, it would mean calling it a day on the world-record attempt. It wasn't a difficult choice to make – there was no way an injured arm was going to stop me.

'I'm fairly confident it's not broken,' I told Becky and the rest of the crew. 'I can keep running. It hurts like hell, but so does everything else. I can handle it.'

Although they were concerned, they could see from the determination on my face there was no point arguing with me as my mind was made up. I was glad they trusted me and supported my decision to carry on. I started running again even though the pain in my arm was excruciating.

I tried to focus on other things. I knew a group of friends were planning to meet me at my next stop at Chepstow Racecourse so I focused on getting there. As I got nearer, a car drove past me tooting its horn and stopped a few yards further on. To my delight, I saw my friends Kate De Haan and Pam Watts get out to give me a hug. They had come all the way from Kent to see me. It was such a welcome distraction from the pain in my arm but there was no disguising my discomfort.

'You look awful,' Pam said as she greeted me. 'You look like you need to be in hospital!'

'Well, it's lovely to see you too!' I said, taking her comments in good humour.

They carried on to the racecourse to wait for me with more of my friends and I was so excited about seeing them again, I was able to pick up the pace and arrive slightly ahead of schedule to smiles and hugs all round. I stopped for some food and while I ate the gathered crowd were all very good at not interfering with my routine and just let the crew and I get on with our well-rehearsed pit-stop. They were horrified when they heard about the hit-and-run and Pam, who once worked as a trauma nurse, had a look at my swollen arm. She agreed it didn't appear to be broken, but in any other circumstances, she wouldn't have recommended anyone to run with such an injury.

The original plan had been for some of the group to run the next six miles with me. It was lovely to have company when friends joined me throughout the challenge, but after the day I'd had, I felt on this occasion I would be happier running alone at my own pace. Thankfully they all understood and wished me well as I hit the road again.

On the next section, I would run back into England by running across the Severn Bridge and then skirt around Bristol to spend the night near Congresbury, Somerset. Running over the Severn Bridge was another big boost but I needed all my mental reserves to get me through the final miles that day. My arm was still throbbing, while my legs and feet were in agony. Often when I am struggling in a race, I think about my family to distract myself from the pain. I thought about Tim, and how marvellously he was doing as part of the crew and how he seemed to be enjoying the experience; I thought about my children, who had been constantly sending me their well-wishes and saying how much they loved and believed in me; I thought of my parents, who couldn't be more proud of how their daughter had become an accomplished ultrarunner after beating an eating disorder.

Sadly, my father hadn't lived to see me do JOGLE as he had passed away the year before. I missed him so much, but running had helped me cope with my grief. When I was running, I felt as though he was with me. When it got tough – like it was now coming to the end of the tenth day of the world-record attempt – I would hear his voice in my head giving me a kick up the backside.

My father's death was the saddest and most painful moment of my life and it happened when I couldn't have been more removed from my family. At the time, I was facing another test of my strength and endurance by taking part in the 6633 Arctic Ultra, a 352-mile non-stop self-sufficiency race held in the Arctic over eight days. It was set up by a friend I had met through ultrarunning called Martin Like and his company, Likeys. He had been planning it for some time and told me to look out for the announcement about the inaugural race in 2007, as he knew I wouldn't want to miss it. He was right, when I heard what was involved, I knew I had to do it.

The race would start at Eagle Plane in the Yukon, cross into the Arctic Circle and then follow the ice road (the frozen Mackenzie River) for 120 miles to eventually finish in Tuktoyaktuk on the frozen Arctic Ocean in the Northwest Territories – right on the edge of polar bear country. Competitors weren't allowed to have their own crew travel alongside them but had to pull everything they needed themselves in a sledge. Daily temperatures would plunge to −40°C, but thanks to the wind chill, which we would face head-on in one section affectionately known as 'Hurricane Alley', it could feel like −70°C.

After Badwater and the MDS, I knew I could run in the extreme heat, but could I run in the extreme cold? I couldn't wait to find out, so I signed up as soon as the entries opened. The race excited me so much that I didn't stop to consider the costs involved. It would set me back several thousand pounds once I'd paid for the flights and all the kit and equipment I would need to survive in the Arctic. But I just knew it was an event that had to be done; somehow I would find the money. Unfortunately, there would be no chance of recouping any of the cost if I ran well, as in those days, prize money at ultra-races was unheard of. Everyone ran for the enjoyment and love of the sport. They weren't motivated by financial gain. I decided to use the savings in what I'd dubbed my 'running away fund' to pay for it. It would be expensive but what an adventure, unlike anything I had ever experienced before.

Once again, Tim was bemused as to why I would choose to run in such brutal conditions but gave me his full support. Emma and Harri thought I was bonkers, but Ruaraidh thought it sounded amazing and wanted to accompany me. It would make the trip even more expensive but I couldn't think of a better mother–son bonding opportunity.

He had finished college and was in between jobs after qualifying to become a personal trainer. Tim and I were worried he had become a bit aimless, so we thought the trip would be just what he needed: a chance for him to travel and see a part of the world few people ever have the privilege to go to. I rang Martin who was more than happy to have Ruaraidh as part of the support crew that travelled with the organisers between checkpoints, helping out by collecting wood, lighting fires and supporting all the competitors.

With the travel plans in place, that just left me to prepare for what was in store on the Arctic expedition. I carried on with my usual long-distance training but started taking a tyre with me. People must have thought I had gone mad when they saw me running through the Kent countryside with the contraption attached to my waist, but I had to get used to running with a weight. During the race, I would be allowed to leave a change of clothes at two checkpoints and at the finish, but everything else I needed for the entire journey I would have to pull along myself in my trusty sledge. It was very important I knew exactly where each item of kit was in my sledge, so I spent a few weeks beforehand strategically planning where everything would be packed. This way, if I needed to stop during the race to find anything, there would be no time wasted rummaging to find it, reducing the risk of getting hypothermia when standing around in the freezing cold.

I was warned everything in the Arctic had to be done as quickly and efficiently as possible – including going to the loo! The sledge needed to be kept as light as possible while still containing everything I would need – food and snacks, a cooking stove with gas cylinders (which had to be wrapped in a pair of ski socks to stop them getting too cold), a full change of clothes and a head torch with a remote battery pack that must be kept under my clothing when worn to protect it from the freezing temperature so it would work. Finally, I needed a 'sleeping bag system'.

This was made up of a sleeping bag with a protection rating against cold temperatures as low as –40°C, with a thin thermal mat placed inside for added warmth. All this would go inside a waterproof bivvy bag and be placed on another more substantial sleeping mat that could be placed on the snow. The 'sleeping system' had to be placed at the top of the sledge so I could quickly grab it to lay it on the snow so I could climb in to the sleeping bag to have a nap during the run if needed. A fellow athlete who had done similar races before gave me a great bit of advice before I left about sleeping during the race. He told me before going to sleep, to always remember to point my sledge in the direction I wanted to go when waking – as the landscape looks so similar. Otherwise I could wake up and run the wrong way!

The right kit was essential. The saying 'fail to prepare then prepare to fail' couldn't be truer when it comes to this race. It wouldn't only be the difference between finishing and not finishing, but in avoiding a stay in hospital with hypothermia or losing a body part to frostbite. Having talked to a lot of people who had taken part in similar events, I was told that layering was the way to go in order to regulate my body temperature. It was extremely important I didn't sweat as this can lead to hypothermia if the sweat cools the body down too much and makes it freeze.

On my top half, I would wear a sports bra, base layer, merino wool fleece, a lined gilet, a wind-proof jacket, and when it got very cold, another thicker down-lined jacket over that. Covering my legs was much simpler. I'd run in thick running tights that were fleece-lined with another pair of fleece-lined, wind-proof trousers over the top so my legs would never get cold. The trousers had zips all the way up the legs allowing them to be easily taken off and on without having to remove my shoes. On my feet, I'd wear a pair of thermal socks, with a thicker pair of winter trekking socks over the top and water-resistant trail shoes to provide extra grip in the snow and keep my feet dry. These were a size larger than I would normally wear to accommodate the thick socks. No part of my face could be exposed due to the risk of frostbite, which meant wearing a rather fetching windstopper hat with flaps to cover my ears, buffs around my neck that could be pulled up over my face and ski goggles to protect my eyes. My fingers would be at a great risk of frostbite and I was particularly concerned about keeping them warm, as they are always the first part of my body to feel the cold. I had three pairs of gloves to wear at the same time – one thin, thermal pair, another slightly thicker set and over them both, a pair of Arctic mitts.

While the majority of what I needed would be packed into my sledge, the items I would need easy access to would be carried around my waist in a bum bag. I filled it with my delicious homemade trail mix – a combination of foods high in carbs, protein and sugar. It was thousands of calories containing raisins, mixed dried fruits such as cranberries, blueberries and sultanas, chopped nuts, dates and crunchy granola. I was delighted to be able to include lots of chocolate – a treat I couldn't carry in hot races as it would melt. There would be no danger of that in the Arctic. To add a bit of variety and extra protein, I also carried pepperoni sausage. I'd have to carry water in a hydration pack underneath my base-layer top to prevent the liquid from freezing. I had to get used to running with it when training, including practising blowing the water back down the pipe after I'd had a sip, as any left in the hose could freeze and block the tube.

I knew this race would be the ultimate test of my physical and mental capabilities. Not just because of the distance I had to run but because of the inhospitable terrain, the biting cold and the remote landscape I would have to navigate alone. With the training done and my kit all prepared, I felt I was as ready as I would ever be. But three weeks before I was due to leave, I received a phone call from my mother which I had been dreading. My father had recently been diagnosed with bladder cancer; his condition had started deteriorating rapidly and he'd been taken into hospital. I arranged to fly up to Edinburgh straightaway to be with him.

Seeing him in his hospital bed was heart-wrenching. He looked a shadow of his former self, but still had his wonderful smile. His weight had plummeted as he had lost his appetite and found eating too painful; all he could manage was jelly. The doctors told my mother, Jacqui and I that as his cancer was terminal and particularly aggressive, he wouldn't have long to live. Hearing this, my mind was made up about the Arctic race: I couldn't go now. When I told my mother and Jacqui, they urged me to reconsider.

'Your father has been so excited hearing about you going to do this race, you have to do it,' my mother told me. 'We are going to follow you online; it will take his mind off the pain hearing about your progress and thinking about how you are getting on. He'll be so proud of you.'

When my father was well enough to talk to me he said the same thing. He wanted me to go and take part in the race. He was proud of everything I had achieved so far and he loved the fact his daughter was now taking on such a massive and extraordinary challenge. His illness proved that life was too short not to pursue your dreams, try new experiences and strive to be your best. He wanted me to go and run it for him. How could I say no?

I spent as much time with him as I could before it was time for me to leave. The last occasion I saw him was on the Sunday before I flew home, a week before I headed out to the Arctic. I spent the morning by his bedside chatting to him, and before I knew it, it was time to leave to catch my flight. As I said goodbye, I gave him the biggest hug I could, terrified I might break his ribs as he was so thin. I told him I loved him and as I walked away I just wanted to cry. Before I went round the corner, I turned to take one last look at him. He was smiling back at me with his beautiful, piercing blue eyes, the love he had for me shining out of his face. It was as if he knew we wouldn't see each other again.

I fought back tears as I walked towards the car; I knew that could have been the last time I would see him alive. The pain was unbearable. All I wanted to do was turn back and give him another hug. Leaving to catch my flight was one of the toughest moments of my life.

Once back at home, my father was still at the forefront of my mind, but I tempered my sadness with resolve. He wanted to see me finish this ultra, so with all the strength and determination I had, I would give it my all. Not only did I want to finish, I had another goal. I wanted to win. Not to be first female, but to do a Pam Reed and win the whole thing outright. Tim stifled a laugh when I told him about the plan but if I could stick to my intended pace and not have too many sleeping breaks, I would be in with a chance. Having completed Badwater in 2005, my confidence was high and I had gone on to complete various ultras where I had managed to finish first female and highly placed overall. One of these races had been another desert ultra – the Kalahari Augrabies Extreme Marathon   a 155-mile self-sufficiency desert race over seven days. I finished first female and sixth overall, an achievement I was particularly pleased with given an exchange that had occurred when I registered for my place at the hotel before the start. Ultrarunning was such a male-dominated sport back then and I always made an effort to look feminine. I didn't want to be 'one of the boys', I wanted to show what girls can do. So the volunteers manning the registration desk looked taken aback by my appearance when I arrived to collect my number wearing a skirt and a pink top with make-up on and a few bangles jangling on my wrist.

'Are you sure you're in the right place?' one of them asked me.

'Perhaps I should have signed up for a cruise instead!' I joked, brushing aside the implied insult. I knew the next day my running would do the talking. I hoped to prove this at the Arctic race too. I believed if I could run well in the cold conditions, I was capable of beating both the female and male competitors alike.

Arriving at Whitehorse, Yukon, for the race, it wasn't just cold, it was freezing. I stepped off the plane into a snowy, icy, Narnia-like landscape, with whiteness as far as the eye could see. The air was so cold on my face, it made my nose go numb. The next few days were spent going over safety briefings and checking all competitors had the correct kit. We had to do some test runs in our racing gear and prove we were capable of lighting our stoves without assistance – they didn't want anyone to be stuck in the middle of the frozen nowhere alone and be unable to boil water.

Everyone was then driven 500 miles north to Eagle Plane, to stay at the only hotel for miles around, which was usually only used to accommodating the ice road truckers. It was full of them when we arrived as they had been stranded due to the bad weather over the past three days. It was such a blizzard, even the snowplough drivers had to wait for the weather to improve to get out and clear the way. They were all killing time over a few drinks at the hotel bar and enjoyed the distraction of hearing about our race when we arrived. They were used to crossing the wintry tundra in their lorries and couldn't believe we were mad enough to run across it.

I hadn't intended to join them in the bar the night before the race (I had learned my lesson from the Grand Union Canal Race!), but I didn't have any choice when I found out my sledge was going to need some modification. Due to all the grit that had been put down on the roads for the truckers to drive safely, our sledges would need wheels or they would get damaged. The hotel manager had attempted to help me attach the wheels to mine, but one of the mechanisms wasn't working properly. The sledge kept tipping forwards and dragging on the ground. There was no way I could race with it like that, so I had to brave the testosterone-filled bar and ask if any of the truckers had a toolkit in their lorry I could borrow. They were pretty pissed at this point, so explaining what I needed was particularly difficult, especially as they couldn't believe a 'little lady' like me was planning to do the 'crazy' race they had heard so much about. Thankfully, one of the truckers eventually lent me his box of tools and between me and some of the other racers we managed to sort my sledge out. I finally got to bed at midnight.

The following morning, two hours later than originally planned due to the bad weather, the race could begin. I joined the other ten runners and a couple, Denise and Jon Whyte, who intended to cycle the course on a tandem (yes, a tandem – and I thought I was mad!) on the start line, a short stroll from the hotel. Decked out in my Arctic attire with my sledge around my waist, I set out into the white wilderness. We ran along an undulating road of compacted snow through a forest of snow-capped trees and across a bridge over the fast-flowing Yukon River, with the Richardson Mountains in view to our right. The sun was just coming up in the pale blue sky with the rays bouncing off the snow. We were running in a winter wonderland.

It wasn't long before the small field spread out and I found myself at the front being chased by one man. I hadn't expected to take the lead so soon but I didn't panic, I knew I just had to stick to my original race plan. The first checkpoint was at 23 miles, where we would then cross into the Arctic Circle – a great photo opportunity as you can pose beside a giant wooden information board with the sign *Arctic Circle Lat 66° 33'N*. As we approached this checkpoint, the organisers were taking bets on who would get there first. My lovely son hadn't backed me, so you can imagine his total surprise when he saw his mother arrive first. The weather had remained so bad, the authorities had said no one could pass beyond the Arctic Circle that day as it was dangerous. The organisers said we must all return to the hotel for the night, and then be driven back to the first checkpoint the following day to continue our journey. I was disappointed as I was feeling good and wanted to carry on while I was in the groove, but safety had to come first.

The following morning, the race was back on and we could enter the Arctic Circle, running on to reach the section known as Hurricane Alley, and boy, did it live up to its name. At their strongest, the winds along this road can overturn a lorry. I was buffeted all over the place and had to bend forward with my head down in order to keep moving onwards. I was glad of my sledge anchoring me to the ground; without it, I feared I could have been blown away. The biting wind swirled snow into my face and it was hard to see where I was going. When I went to take a sip of water in my hydration pack, I discovered the cold combined with the wind chill had caused the liquid to freeze. I was going to have to run the next few miles thirsty as I didn't want to stop to melt water to drink on my stove.

Despite wearing my three pairs of gloves, my hands felt like blocks of ice. It was hard to know how far I had run as my watch was hidden beneath all my layers so it was impossible to check it. It was the same for the mp3 player I was wearing, which I quickly realised was a bad idea to run with here. If it played a song I didn't want to listen to, I couldn't skip to the next track as there was no chance of reaching the gadget submerged in my clothing.

When I finally reached the support vehicle, which was waiting at the end of Hurricane Alley, Martin, the race director, told me that with the wind chill, the temperature had plummeted to –70°C. No wonder I had lost all sensation in the tips of my fingers! There would be a chance to warm up at the next stop, as every checkpoint had some form of shelter to offer a bit of respite from the wind and cold. These might be sheds usually used for ice fishing or log cabins belonging to local Inuit. At one of the checkpoints, known as Swimming Pool Point, there was nothing but a caravan that looked as though it had been abandoned in the middle of nowhere after someone had run out of petrol. I was glad of every checkpoint, not only as it offered the chance to warm up slightly but because I could check how Ruaraidh was doing. He thought I was crazy when I asked him to wake me up after just two hours' sleep when I met him at the second checkpoint, but I knew I had to stick to my plan.

When he woke me up, it was incredibly difficult to get out of my snuggly sleeping bag. I longed to stay tucked up in my warm bed rather than go out running in the freezing cold. But I knew I had to force myself up if I was going to win, giving me the motivation to get out of my cosy bed. After having something to eat, I was soon running again – my entire break only amounting to four hours, while my male rival slumbered on.

It was another 47 miles to the next checkpoint and now I had dropped the other leading runner, it meant covering this distance completely alone – except on the instances when the race organisers would drive by to check I was OK. There was never any danger of getting lost as there was only one road cut through the snow, I just had to keep going in the same direction.

Running alone surrounded by snow and ice was mentally challenging but I really enjoyed the solitude. There were no ringing phones, no blaring televisions and no children asking me to do something for them. The only noise was the sound of my breathing and of my feet crunching on the snow. Luckily for me, there was also no one around to complain about my singing as I sang at the top of my voice to pass the time after giving up on my mp3 player. Of course, I thought I sounded amazing. The wind had dropped, making it beautifully calm and still, giving me the time (when I wasn't singing to myself) to take in the peace and tranquillity of my majestic surroundings. I passed a frozen lake that sparkled with the most magnificent shade of blue – a colour I had never seen before or since – and crested snowy hills that afforded a spectacular view of the white plains stretching out beneath me. Another highlight was when twilight arrived and the sky lit up with the phenomenal Northern Lights. It was awe-inspiring to see the kaleidoscope of colours above me as I ran and meant on a few occasions I had no need to wear a head torch as they lit my way through the darkness.

At each checkpoint, the organisers told me I was pulling further and further ahead of the other runners. This meant my running solitude would continue for the rest of the race, just me and the miles and miles of snow. Racing such a long distance on very little sleep was exhausting and around 200 miles in to the race, just before the Caribou Creek checkpoint, I lost about half an hour as a result. I woke up with a start to discover I had fallen asleep standing up, only managing to stay upright thanks to my sledge. Feeling bleary eyed as I resumed my solitary run in the remote, endlessly white environment, my mind started playing tricks on me and I started to have hallucinations. At least, I know now they were hallucinations – at the time they seemed completely real. Cartoon characters would elongate in front of me and as I got closer to them, they'd pop up as if they were going to hit me on the nose. Next, I saw an elephant sitting on a bridge. I then began seeing hundreds of men either side of me wearing white Arctic suits and black gas masks, sitting on snowmobiles and carrying guns, looking as though they were about to attack. Further along the road I saw a whole troop of them beside vehicles forming a blockade. I had to close my eyes, count to ten and tell myself they weren't really there, it was all only in my weird and wonderful imagination.

When I reached the next checkpoint, I told Ruaraidh and the doctor about my hallucinations, causing the doctor to be extremely concerned for me, especially when I told her I was only planning to rest for a couple of hours. She told me quite firmly that I shouldn't carry on until I'd had at least six hours' sleep.

'I can't sleep for that long, I can only have four-hour breaks if I want to win,' I told her.

Martin told me I could have ten hours' sleep and I would still win by miles, as I was that far ahead of anyone else. But I was so tired I couldn't get my head around what they were saying. Only my original plan made any sense to me; I felt if I deviated from it, I would lose. In a reversal of our past roles, Ruaraidh took control and picked me up and carried me to a bed where I fell straight to sleep. I woke up two hours later to find I was surrounded by a group of Inuit who were staring at me as though I had landed there from another planet. It was most peculiar, and this time I wasn't hallucinating!

After my sleep, I ate some food and was then back on my way – resting for five hours in total in the end. The Northern Lights lit up the sky again as I ran. This time one of the rays swooshed around me, then went in a big loop until it appeared to be going at the same pace as me on my right hand side. The beautiful light looked like a smiley face with eyes and an upturned mouth and a bowler hat on. As the flume of green light continued to run alongside me, I felt as though it was trying to tell me something but I couldn't work out what it was. I even started talking to it but of course I received no reply and it eventually swooshed off into the distance, leaving me alone once more with my own thoughts. The next checkpoint was the Arctic Chalets 30 miles away and I kept focusing on getting there by putting one foot in front of the other. Not only did I long for the roaring log fires I knew would be waiting for me there, it was the only spot on the entire course with Wi-Fi. I usually avoid checking my emails during a race so I can concentrate on the job in hand but I needed to find out how my father was. When I logged on at the blessed checkpoint, it was lovely to get an email from my mother who wrote that she and my father had been following my progress online and were both so proud of me. She had told me matter-of-factly before I had left that she wouldn't tell me mid-race if my father had died as 'there isn't anything you can do about it', but I knew she wouldn't have lied and mentioned him if it wasn't true. I felt so relieved.

After a short break, I began my journey on the next section of the race – the long ice road – feeling invigorated by my mother's email – my father was still alive and tracking my run. However, about two minutes after leaving the Arctic Chalets, a feeling of devastation washed over me. I felt as though I had been punched in the heart and I couldn't breathe. A huge sense of loss overwhelmed me and I knew that my father had passed away. It was as if I could feel his presence, as though he had come to see me to tell me himself. I can't explain why I felt so certain about it, but I knew that was the moment my father had died.

I considered turning back so I could check my emails again, but I knew there was little point as my mother wouldn't confirm the devastating news till I had finished. My chin trembled as I struggled to stop myself sobbing but I couldn't hold back the tears as they started to roll down my face in an endless stream, my heart was broken. I began talking to my father: 'This is so not a good time to die,' I told him. 'I can't cry here as my tears will freeze.'

I had no choice but to keep on going. Four hours later one of the support vehicles passed me and I solemnly told Martin, when he checked how I was, that I was certain that my father had died.

'You can't be sure of that,' he replied. 'Try not to worry.'

But I was adamant. It was only later that I discovered I was right. My father had indeed died at the exact time I had headed out on the ice road.

I couldn't give in to my grief then as I knew the final 120 miles of the race would be the greatest test of my mental resilience. I would need all my strength and determination to get by running alone along the remainder of the ice road – aka the Mackenzie River. It was surreal to run on the frozen river, the compacted ice shimmered in stunning shades of blue, yellow and green beneath my feet. I was slightly concerned with the amount of cracks I could see. I kept worrying that I might fall through into the icy waters below. The sound of it creaking under my feet brought back memories of the time Jacqui fell through thin ice in Norway, which I quickly tried to push away again. I had to keep reassuring myself that if the ice road could take the weight of lorries driven by the truckers, it would certainly stay in one piece for me.

This section of the race was the most challenging as the frozen river ran in a very long, straight path through incredibly monotonous scenery. Aside from the glimmering frozen river beneath my feet, everything else around and above me was white, as if I was running across a blank page. There were no landmarks around to judge how far I had run and there was nothing up ahead to aim for. It was just a case of keeping moving through the whiteness with no end in sight. The ice road stretched out as far as the eye could see.

As I ran on, I became desperate for a pee and knew I wouldn't be able to hold it in till the next checkpoint, which was still many miles away. I was going to have to brave the cold to go. As there was no one else around I thought it would be safe just to quickly squat on the side of the road, I didn't want to venture off track in case I became buried in the snow. I untied my sledge, whipped my mitts and gloves off and pulled down my trousers to relieve myself. As it had been a long time since I had last been, it went on and on, and with typical timing, to my dismay two trucks appeared on the horizon in both directions. I tried to pee faster in a desperate attempt to finish and pull my trousers up before they passed, but to no avail. I had to suffer the embarrassment of being caught with my pants down as the truckers drove past gleefully beeping their horns at me. All I could do was wave back, feeling mortified but seeing the funny side.

After my loo break, as I settled back into my running rhythm, I expected to have nothing but the snow as company again as the trucks moved off into the distance. So I was shocked sometime later when I heard footsteps coming from behind me. I wondered if my mind was playing tricks again and then I started panicking. I knew I shouldn't have rested for so long earlier, now someone was going to overtake me! As the footsteps got louder I could tell by the speed of the approach that whoever they belonged to had much more spring in their step than me, so I wouldn't be able to compete with them. As they drew level I saw it was a French competitor, who I knew had been pulled out of the race much earlier due to suffering from frostbite. It was then I recalled the organisers saying that anyone who was pulled out of completing the full race could rejoin for the final section if they had recovered – although of course they would not be eligible for a medal or able to share the glory of completing the full event. So my French companion was not a rival but enjoying a run on the last part of the course. It was nice to have a running buddy but we soon discovered we wouldn't be able to have a conversation as he had no English and I can't speak French.

The last checkpoint was the caravan in the middle of the snowy wilderness at Swimming Pool Point. By the time I got there, my shoe laces had frozen so they couldn't be untied. I had to curl up for a nap in my sleeping bag with them still on. Luckily I had been warned this could happen so I had packed plastic bags to put over them first so I wouldn't get my sleeping bag wet.

When I awoke, I felt buoyant. I was now only 45 miles from the finish and still miles out in the lead. It looked as though I was going to achieve my goal – I was actually going to win the race. I resumed running, alone again as the Frenchman opted for a longer rest, but I didn't mind as it allowed me to soak up my amazing surroundings, knowing this was the last time I would be running here. The sun rose, creating a glorious pink sky against the white landscape. It was one of the most beautiful things I had ever seen and I knew I had to stop to take the panoramic scene in and commit it to my memory. I wanted to mark the moment but as I didn't have a camera, I decided to take off my sledge and then use my feet to write out the word *MARVELLOUS* in giant letters in the snow.

When I started running again, my good mood could almost have been my downfall as I misjudged the distance to the finish. I could see the lights of the town of Tuktoyaktuk – the final destination – twinkling in the distance and I picked up my pace, galvanised by the fact the finish was now in sight. The increase in pace meant I dangerously started sweating. I

WINNING AND LOSING IN THE ARCTIC

told myself it didn't matter as there were only a few miles left and then I would be able to change into some warm clothes. I hadn't realised there were still about 16 miles to go. As I carried on running, the sky behind me suddenly lit up and I was sure it was one of the support vehicles approaching with their headlights on. I turned back to see it was actually the spectacular colours of the Northern Lights, coming out to play one last time.

When Ruaraidh and the race organisers did catch up with me to check on my progress, I had expected it to be the fantastic moment they would direct me to the finish line. Instead they joyfully told me I 'only had six miles to go'. I felt like bursting into tears. They thought hearing the short distance left would be music to my ears, but after running for days in the freezing cold, the thought of another six miles when I had been convinced I was nearly finished seemed impossible. I felt absolutely frozen and was shivering uncontrollably. I was already wearing all the clothes I had and was worried I wouldn't make it to the finish in this condition. From inside the support vehicle, one of my fellow competitors, who had been pulled out of the race earlier and was getting a lift, kindly offered to lend me his hat and padded jacket. I now had so many layers on I looked like the Michelin Man, but at least I was beginning to feel warm again.

Ruaraidh noticed how much I was struggling and asked if he could join me for the final six-mile run in. It wasn't against the rules as long as he didn't give me any assistance such as by pulling my sledge for me. His company made all the difference although he probably regretted joining me as I couldn't stop moaning and groaning about how slow I was going and how we didn't seem to be making any progress.

'It's still so far away! The town isn't getting any closer!' I kept complaining. 'I actually think it is getting further away!'

'Don't be silly,' he replied. 'Look, the roofs are getting much bigger.'

He must have thought I had completely lost the plot when I insisted I could see a ballerina dancing in the snow and was frustrated when he couldn't see her also.

'Look, she's right there!' I kept saying pointing to my hallucination.

I then attempted to do a faster run to try to end the ordeal earlier but Ruaraidh pointed out I was actually going quicker by power walking instead of jogging due to being weighed down by all my layers, so we plodded purposefully on with Ruaraidh telling me numerous stories to take my mind off my pain.

The town of Tuktoyaktuk was now definitely getting closer. At 5.30 a.m., we finally reached it. Despite the early hour, all the locals had come out to greet me and were clapping and cheering as I made my way through the streets towards the finish line between two igloos on the frozen Arctic Ocean. It was an amazing end to what had been a spectacular race.

I was overcome with emotion as I crossed the finish line, giving my son a huge hug – I had done it. I had achieved my goal – I had won overall. As it was the inaugural race, my time of 143 hours 23 minutes (completed in just under six days) was a course record – and at the time of writing, it is yet to be broken. I felt so proud; it had all been worthwhile: this one was for my father.

It felt marvellous to remove the sledge from my waist and change into warm, dry clothing. As soon as I could I found a telephone and called home. I was devastated when my mother confirmed what I had already suspected, that my father had died.

'He was so proud of you,' my mother told me through tears, 'we all are.'

My mother told me one comfort had been that my father had been allowed to leave hospital a few days before he passed away so he was able to fulfil his wish to die peacefully at home. The day he left hospital was when I had seen that smiley face in the Northern Lights, I felt that's what it had been trying to tell me as it had made me feel content. After I spoke to my mother I was heartbroken and so glad Ruaraidh was with me so we could support one another in our grief. He was close to his grandfather and was devastated by his loss. It was hard being so far away from the rest of our family at this time but I couldn't have any regrets about making the trip. My father had wanted me to race and I had emphatically won in his memory.

The scale of my achievement soon became evident, as it was another 24 hours till the next competitor – Steve Evans – came in. Of the 12 competitors who had started, seven had been forced to withdraw and the other three finishers, including my rival who had chased me at the start, finished outside the eight-day limit. Meanwhile, Denise and Jon completed the course on their tandem, which was an incredible feat.

It was a wonderful feeling being able to tell people 'I won' when they asked how the race went. The best reaction was when we encountered the ice road truckers again as we celebrated back at the hotel.

'So, who won?' they said, looking at the men when we walked in. Their jaws hit the floor when my fellow competitors pointed to me. Then one of them brought me back down to earth when he quipped: 'Aren't you the one we saw having a pee on the ice road?'

Back at home, it was an incredibly difficult time as I grieved for my father. I was reduced to floods of tears when I read a race report online, penned by Martin, in which he spoke so kindly about me. He wrote:

Mimi continues to be inspirational. For anyone who doesn't know Mimi, let me try to briefly describe this barking mad woman. She is as slight as any person I can imagine, she loves pink, she is absolutely driven and she has been the topic of conversation amongst everyone involved in the race. She is living proof that in extreme ultra-distance racing women can be men's equal and in this case can quite possibly kick ass too.

They were such lovely words, I knew my father would have been incredibly proud.

CHAPTER SIX

A RACE AGAINST TIME TO RUN INTO THE RECORD BOOKS

Day 11: Congresbury to North Tawton, 65 miles

Waking up on day 11 of JOGLE in Somerset I felt absolutely shattered. My whole body was aching, particularly my bruised and battered arm, and I just couldn't face getting out of bed, let alone running all day. As always, Becky woke me up with a smoothie and a coffee at 4.30 a.m. She had been up before me to get my drinks ready without fail every day and I couldn't have been more grateful as I knew she wasn't usually a morning person. After she left the drinks by my bedside I thought to myself 'just five more minutes' and dozed off again. Five minutes turned into ten minutes, then 15.

'Come on, Mimi, you have to get up now!' Becky came back and told me, sounding like a mother trying to get a teenager out of bed to go to school. Every morning she had managed to get me up and running by 5 a.m. and she was determined this morning would be no different. But I simply couldn't muster the energy or motivation to get out of bed. All I wanted to do was sleep. In the end, Becky had to help me get dressed and miraculously I still managed to haul my exhausted body out the motorhome door to start running on schedule. Alan normally joined me for the first run of the day but this morning Tim had volunteered to take his place, allowing Alan time to catch up on some much-needed extra sleep. My poor husband probably ended up regretting this decision as I was in a foul mood. For the whole four hours till the next rest stop, all I could do was gripe about how exhausted I was and how slow I was moving. I grumbled and groaned non-stop, nothing positive came out of my mouth.

'What's the point? I'm not going to get the record as I'm going too slowly,' I complained. 'Everything hurts so much, I can't run, I'm not going to do this.'

Moan, moan, moan. Perhaps if Alan rather than my husband had been with me I wouldn't have gone on quite so much and I would have tried to be more positive. But as it was Tim I didn't hold back and I kept whinging on and on as he cycled beside me. He was brilliant and extremely patient; he didn't interrupt but just gave the odd grunt. Eventually he turned and said to me: 'Mimi, no one is making you do this. You can stop at any time. But if you do, just think how you will feel tomorrow.'

He was right. I was being defeatist and I knew I wasn't going to quit. Perhaps I had just needed a good vent, as I felt so much better having ranted and moaned for hours (poor Tim). He went on ahead as we approached our first break of the day – no doubt to warn the others how negative I was feeling. When I arrived, Phil presented me with a bowl of porridge with a strawberry lovingly placed in the middle, how could I be grumpy now? Becky and Alan had my stats on the last four hours. Becky told me how many miles I had run and I was amazed. It was much further than I thought considering how bad I felt. I had assumed my battered and weary body had only managed a couple of miles in four hours, so I feared I was completely off target.

'You're making good progress,' Becky told me as she gave my legs a quick massage. 'You are a little bit down on where you need to be at this point but not much, you can make it up later in the day. Of course you are going to be tired. It isn't going to feel as easy as it did at the start but you just have to keep going – you're doing really well.'

The warming porridge, a strong coffee and Becky's pep talk was the perfect remedy and in the next four-hour running stint I was in a much happier frame of mind. It brought home to me just how important the crew are when doing a challenge like this one. They all said and did exactly the right thing to give me a boost and keep me going. Too much sympathy would have made me feel sorry for myself and more likely to quit. And if they had risen to my moaning and become angry about it, I could have forced them to walk out and leave me to it, as I must have seemed so ungrateful. Instead they were calm, patient and reminded me of my goal and why I was doing this – for a world record. I was learning that achieving it would take as much mental resilience as physical hardship – this was unlike anything I had done before. It wasn't like a race where you had other runners to compete against, I was running alone against the clock. As a record was at stake, maintaining a decent pace was paramount. If I had a bad patch, I couldn't afford to stop until I felt better, I had to keep going. I couldn't let the goal slip from my mind and I couldn't doubt my ability to do it as I had done earlier in the day. If I started believing I wasn't going to get the record, then it would be easy to stop – what would have been the point in carrying on? The moment doubt begins to creep into your mind, it is the beginning of the end so such thoughts have to be banished before they can take hold. I had to stay focused.

Reaching Land's End was not the goal, getting there in record time was. Keeping this in mind empowered me to keep putting one foot in front of the other and banish all the moaning, negative thoughts from my mind. My rant had been cathartic. I felt now I had said all I needed to, it was out of my system and I could carry on and be positive. It helped that we were now getting closer to Becky and Phil's home turf in Cornwall. There was no chance we were going to get lost now as they knew the roads we were travelling along inside out. They could guide me with ease through the towns, point out local landmarks and prewarn me of any big hills coming up (of which there seemed to be a lot in Devon!).

Although they didn't let their concerns be known to me at the time for fear of disheartening me after my morning meltdown, the crew were beginning to worry about how much further from the target pace I was, as my fatigue was forcing me to run more slowly and have longer walking breaks. Tim and Alan had been regularly checking the maps and cross-referencing everything to ensure we were still on record time but it was now getting tighter and tighter.

That night after we had parked up on the outskirts of Dartmouth National Park and I had gone to bed, Tim, Becky and Phil stayed up to discuss what could be done, allowing Alan to go to bed so he could be up to cycle the first early shift with me. They realised if we stuck to the current plan, I wasn't going to make it to Land's End in time. Despite the fact they were all exhausted and would have to be up again in a few hours, they battled their drooping eyelids to determine a new schedule to help me obtain the record. They realised rest periods were going to have to be stripped back further on days 12 and 13. I wouldn't be able to stop for lunch any more but would have to eat while on the move. At the end of day 12, I'd only be able to have two hours' sleep instead of four. With the plan in place, they finally hit the sack.

Day 12: Crediton to Bodmin, 61 miles

I stirred at 4.30 a.m. feeling confused when I checked the time as there was no sign nor any sound from the rest of the motorhome. Where was Becky? She was so tired after their late night planning the new schedule she'd overslept. Luckily, my body clock had intervened. Becky flew into a panic when it was me who woke her up, but there was no harm done and I was back running as normal by 5 a.m., with an exhausted Alan taking on the cycling duties. He explained the new plan letting me know that from now on, I was going to have fewer rest stops and a shorter sleep that night. I didn't complain or question him, if the crew thought that was the best way for me to get the record then I was going to listen and obey, I completely trusted their judgement. Alan told me that as tired as I was, I had to try to maintain a decent pace, even when walking. As he cycled behind me, he offered words of encouragement to keep me in a rhythm and focused on my running action.

'Stride with purpose!' he'd tell me. 'Don't shuffle!'

I don't know how but I managed to keep lifting one foot in front of the other even though my whole body was in agony. I just kept focusing on the finish. There was a treat in store to raise my spirits as the crew completely spoilt me for lunch. Becky and Phil knew of a fish-and-chip shop near Okehampton so stopped as we passed to buy some for us. They were the most marvellous fish and chips I have ever tasted. I was in heaven. I'm not normally one for savouring my food but this meal was delicious and divine, just what I needed to get me through the rest of the day. Who needs Michelin-starred restaurants when you can have perfectly battered fish and chips?

We continued along the A30 with Becky taking her turn on the bike behind me. With the fish and chips in my stomach and the sun shining, I was feeling much more positive, even managing to ignore any pain as we passed a sign that said, *Welcome to Cornwall.* This was a huge moment for me. Since the challenge had begun, I had run through three countries (Scotland, England and Wales) and 19 counties including the Highlands, Cumbria, Herefordshire and Somerset. Leaving Devon behind meant I was entering the final county. I could finally start counting down the miles to the finish, which were now in double rather than treble digits – just 70 to go until the running would stop. The end was in sight. As I passed the sign, Becky shouted to me: 'Lift your arms up, Mimi, in celebration of entering Cornwall!'

Although I was exhausted, I felt elated in the moment and mustered the energy to raise my arms to the sky. Becky snapped a photo from behind me and then I heard her in a fit of giggles: she'd nearly fallen off the bike as she'd taken the shot but thankfully it was just a wobble.

I ploughed on with minimal breaks, eating as I ran along the A30 surrounded by mostly slow-moving traffic. It was a special day for Phil and Becky as we were now passing through their home county. Becky met up with her mother at Launceston, who came armed with a delicious and very much-appreciated chicken casserole, while Phil's wife later paid us a visit. Phil's friends Glynn Griffen and Paul George also made the effort to come and support us. Paul and Becky would go on to marry in the future, but that's another story! Seeing the new faces gave everyone a much-needed boost and the day passed by smoothly, with only one moment of panic when Phil thought he'd lost the keys to one of the motorhomes.

Finally, it was time for me to go to bed but with only two hours' sleep, it felt as though I was up and running again before my head had even hit the pillow.

Day 13: Bodmin to Land's End, 55 miles

Rising for the final day of the challenge was easier than on the previous two days, despite only having had two hours' sleep. I knew this was the final day and I felt excited and anxious at the same time to see what the day would bring – could I get the world record? If I could use every last ounce of energy I had left to keep going for another 55 miles, then I would find out.

Alan was awake and ready to accompany me on the bike, while Becky slept in for longer and Tim drove one of the motorhomes, using it to keep leapfrogging my position. Meanwhile, Phil drove on ahead so he could stop and have my porridge ready when I caught up. However, he was so tired when he arrived, he fell asleep in the passenger seat when he pulled over and was alarmed when he was woken up by Tim, who arrived in the other motorhome two hours later.

'Mimi's nearly here!' he told him knocking on the window.

Phil couldn't believe it, he felt as though he had only shut his eyes for a second – the sleep deprivation was taking its toll on all of us.

As the day went on, the new schedule was proving to be a success and thanks to the lack of sleep and meals on the go, I was back within record time. There was an air of positivity among us, I was overcoming my physical and mental barriers. What could stop me now? The answer was the long arm of the law.

Running towards Cambourne in the afternoon, still on the A30 heading towards Land's End, I attracted the attention of a passing police officer, apparently a member of the public had complained about a runner on the road and he had been sent to investigate. He asked the crew in the motorhomes to pull over and told me to stop running as he took out his notepad to ask what we were doing.

'You can't run along a main road the way you are,' he told me. 'It's not safe, you could easily be hit by a car.'

The irony of this wasn't lost on me given I had been struck by a car just days before but I wasn't going to tell him about that. That incident had been down to careless driving and I wasn't concerned it would happen again. (Surely lightning doesn't strike twice?) I was running on the edge of the road decked out in my usual high-vis clothing with a cyclist behind me in similarly bright gear, you couldn't miss us. We were sticking to the Highway Code and as long as cars overtook us with plenty of room, as they should do a cyclist, there was no reason for the officer to stop us. Alan made all these points to the policeman and told him we were on the last leg of our world-record attempt but it all seemed to fall on deaf ears. I left them to it as I didn't have the energy to argue. I made the most of the delay to have a much-needed rest and sat down in the back of the police car as it started to rain.

As the minutes ticked by and the policeman was still insistent we would have to change our route, I became increasingly upset and impatient. I couldn't afford to lose this time and still achieve the record. We couldn't take a different route either, that would take too much time – the diversion the policeman recommended would cost us two hours. I had to keep running along the A30, and I needed to get going again as soon as possible. We had now been held up for more than half an hour and with every second the record was slipping from my reach. I had never felt so low or defeated – after everything I had gone through for the past 12 days, it looked like the record was going to be taken away from me and there was nothing I could do about it. I felt any glimmer of hope there had been that I could still achieve the record had disappeared. All I could see was blackness; the lights had gone out. I got my phone out and sent a text to my great friend Guy Jennings, who lives in South Africa explaining what was going on as my crew continued to argue with the officer.

That's it, I wrote. *I will finish by making it to Land's End but the record has been taken away. I simply can't see how I am going to get it now.*

Guy instantly called me and told me: 'Yes, you will get the record. Treat this as a rest stop, eat, drink and relax and when the policeman lets you, get off your backside and go, you can do this!'

It was exactly what I needed to hear as I was really struggling to stay positive. Becky tried her best to buck me up by reinforcing Guy's words and making sure I ate.

'Just treat this as if it's a planned rest,' she said. 'You can, and will, still do this.'

She was brilliant, completely understanding my feelings of total devastation and continually trying to keep me positive. Finally, the police officer relented and let us continue and I tried to resume running with vigour. The hold-up had cost us 45 minutes but I couldn't panic about that now. I couldn't turn back time or stop the clock, I could only control the present and that meant carrying on running as fast as my exhausted body could manage. However, no matter how hard I tried, and despite my wonderful crew's encouragement, I was finding it a real struggle to get myself motivated again and into a positive mindset. My blistered feet hurt and my muscles had stiffened up after sitting in the police car for so long. I tried all the tricks I knew to try to find some chink of light, anything I could grasp onto that could flick the switch in my brain from negative to positive and get me moving faster. Then it came as we passed a sign that read, *Penzance 13 miles*.

I can do that, I thought. *It's only a half-marathon*.

Luckily in my tired state, it had slipped my mind that I had actually another 11 miles to run beyond Penzance, so it was really closer to a marathon that I had left. But the mistake was the impetus I needed to look on the bright side. The switch in my brain was flicked, the lights were back on. I could still get the record.

Becky, Phil, Tim and Alan took it in turns to run or cycle beside me, continually urging me to keep going and reading out messages that were coming in from the 'real' world. The excitement had been building as followers of my pink dot could see my world-record attempt was on a knife edge. Support was flooding in to my website from friends, family and complete strangers, all caught up in the drama and willing me on. Hearing their words of encouragement was a huge incentive to help me keep pushing on, every single message gave me such a boost and I was overwhelmed by how many people were backing me.

As I hit the final, long stretch of road that would take me to Land's End, I could smell the sea. *Not far to go now*, I thought. It was getting dark and local people who had been following my progress online were starting to overtake to meet me at the end.

'See you at the finish!' they called out through their car windows as they went by. Unbeknown to me at the time, half my village back home in Kent were also following me via the pink tracker – from inside my own house! Ruaraidh had been given strict instructions ('under pain of death', as he put it) not to allow anyone other than a couple of select friends over while Tim and I were away. He claims it is a rule he 'of course stuck to diligently, maintaining a state of constant boredom for nearly all of the eight days you were both away'. But on the final day of the challenge, as he followed my progress via the pink tracker and exchanged messages with Tim, he saw I was within touching distance of the record, and felt he couldn't possibly celebrate his mother's momentous achievement, if I got the record, alone. He invited his friend Ollie over and, beers in hand, they followed the pink dot as it moved slowly closer to Land's End. When the beers ran out, they decided to go to the local pub at the end of our road and asked the landlord to get the tracker up on the pub computer so they could continue to follow my progress.

As the pub got busier as the evening went on, a crowd began to form around the computer wondering what the pink dot on the screen everyone was following was all about. The curiosity around the pink dot spread like wildfire and soon Ruaraidh was telling everyone about his mother's world-record attempt, and how I was on the verge of breaking it if I could reach Land's End around 11 p.m. Ruaraidh was inundated with stories from people who said they had seen sightings of the 'little pink lady' in question running through the village and along local forest trails, sometimes even dragging a car tyre behind her.

'It was very much akin to sightings of the Loch Ness Monster and the Yeti,' he told me later.

As I struggled along the A30, I was of course oblivious to the 'Mimi fever', as Ruaraidh described it, that had taken hold at the local pub and how everyone was on the edge of their seats following the pink tracker. When the pub closed at 10 p.m., it looked like the party was over and they would all have to go their separate ways to follow the end of my run. But Ruaraidh had a better idea. Throwing caution to the wind, he invited everyone back to our house to see it through to the finish. As word of the party got around, the whole pub and most of the inhabitants of the village rocked up at our door, armed with drinks. With Ruaraidh's laptop set up to follow my journey, they drank and were merry as they willed the little pink dot on. Such were the numbers, some spilled out into the garden seeking shelter under umbrellas as it started to rain.

In Cornwall, the rain had stopped and with eight miles to go, Tim was with me on the bike. I wanted him to be by my side for the final section, but he had been warned by the rest of the crew that if he wasn't able to keep me above a certain pace, another member would have to take over. Meanwhile, the others kept leapfrogging ahead to see me at every mile point to the finish in the hope it would be encouraging for me to know every time another mile was down. But I actually found it totally disheartening. Every mile felt such a long way and when I saw them again I would think, *All that time and I have only run a mile.* They sensed my frustration, and as Tim was doing a good job of keeping me going, with three miles to go, they announced they would see me at the finish. They would go on ahead to Land's End so they could be ready and waiting for me to arrive with a tape of pink loo roll held up for me to break.

Even though the finish was now so close, I was getting slower and slower. Tim and I were both exhausted. By now my whole body was swollen and even my face was slightly puffy. My hands looked as though they had been inflated and my feet were two and a half sizes larger than they had been at the start. Then with two miles to go, the heavens opened again and it started pouring with rain. The road quickly turned into a river and as we splashed through the puddles in the dark, with the rain lashing in our faces, we started to feel disorientated. We passed a turning on our left and weren't sure if it was the way we should go to reach Land's End. There were no signposts and although Tim told me it was straight on, I wasn't convinced. This was the worst possible time to have a marital spat over directions. Luckily we spotted someone to ask and he assured us we were heading the right way. Pausing had been a welcome relief so I then tried to find any excuse to stop again, even if just for a second. I'd scratch my leg, adjust my clothing or tie my shoelace, anything in order to give me a moment without the unbearable pain of running. There was now only a mile to go, but I didn't feel I was going to make it. I was soaking wet, absolutely exhausted and everything hurt from head to toe. I couldn't run another step.

'I can't do it,' I told Tim as I came to a halt and swayed by the roadside on my wobbly legs. 'I can't go any further, I'm in so much pain. Please call the crew and tell them to come and pick us up. I can't carry on. It hurts too much.'

'Don't be ridiculous!' he replied, aghast at my decision. 'You can't give up now! Do you realise you are only a mile from the finish? You have run 839 miles, you just need to keep moving and manage another one!'

I know it wasn't rational to have come this far and throw the towel in with such a short distance to go, but it seemed something in my mind was now trying to override the drive that had kept me going for so long. It was listening to my broken body and telling it that running any further was not an option. The instinctive self-preservation within me didn't care about a world record. As far as my body and mind were concerned at that point, I had reached the limit of my endurance. But while I was now ready to give up, Tim wasn't going to let me. He knew the rest of the crew were counting on him to get me to the finish – and that he'd have to live with me and how devastatingly disappointed I'd be if I didn't make it.

'You've come so far, Mimi,' he told me. 'Just one more mile and you could be a world-record holder! One more mile and then you can stop and celebrate and all this will have been worth it.'

Then he added: 'Don't think you can give up now and try again next year as we can't go through all this again!'

I knew he was right. I had come this far and Tim, Becky, Alan, Karyn and Phil had sacrificed so much to help me and pushed their own bodies to the brink of exhaustion. I had to keep moving. If I gave up now, I would regret it for ever and I wouldn't be able to face the disappointment from the others. I had to keep going if not for my sake, then for theirs. They had put their hearts and souls into supporting me. Even if I wasn't going to make it in time to get the record, I had to at least finish after everything we had been through.

Slowly dragging one foot in front of the other, I resumed my plod. It was the longest mile of my life but then through the darkness and the downpour, I could finally see the finish in the glow of the lights from the white Land's End visitors' centre building. There was a crowd gathered under umbrellas holding torches around the painted 'FINISH' sign on the road and a string of (now very soggy) loo paper held up for me to break as I ran through. I don't know where I mustered the energy from given I had nothing left just the mile before but I managed to raise my pace slightly for a sprint finish of sorts. The thought of finishing made all the pain disappear and I felt like I was flying as I crossed the line to a loud cheer from the gathered crowd, which included the local mayor and a friend, Ron Thomas, who had driven all the way from Kent to see me finish. It was 11.03 p.m. when Alan stopped his watch, delighted to tell me I had broken the female world record. I was elated. I had done JOGLE in 12 days, 15 hours, 46 minutes and 35 seconds, beating the previous record by 36 minutes.

As people offered me their congratulations, I felt so emotional. I couldn't believe I had done it. While I wanted to celebrate, I was too exhausted and simply had to sit down, my body was utterly spent. Tim helped me into the motorhome where I changed into dry clothes and Becky gave me a massage. The celebrations continued outside as Becky and I reflected on the journey we had shared over the past 12 days.

'I knew you would do it,' she told me. 'Even after you got hit by a car and stopped by the police!'

Outside the motorhome I heard a champagne cork pop as Tim and the others cracked open a bottle to toast our success. He brought in glasses for Becky and me but I could only manage a sip – most unlike me, but I just couldn't stomach it. Tim received a call on his mobile from Ruaraidh as he and his band of followers had noticed the tracker had reached Land's End and were all now waiting with bated breath as Ruaraidh made the call to hear if I had finished in record time.

'Your mother's done it! She's got the record!' Tim declared, followed by, 'Who are all those people cheering in the background?'

He passed the phone over so Ruaraidh could congratulate me and I could barely hear him as he held up the phone so his assortment of drunken gathered guests could cheer and applaud me. I was stunned when he told me, full of emotion, that the whole village had been cheering me on and sent their best wishes. If I hadn't been so tired, I probably would have told Ruaraidh to make sure they all tidied up before they left but I didn't have the energy and I didn't care. I felt so overwhelmed that my son and so many others had cared about how I had got on.

The tears continued to flow when I received a lovely message from Emma, who had also been keeping a constant eye on the tracker while tending to my three-month-old grandson, Theo. She wrote how they were immensely proud of me and loved me so much, they couldn't wait to see me when I got home.

Harri had no idea at this stage that I had finished as she was on holiday, so I sent her a message to tell her the good news. Meanwhile my amazing mother, who had made it to various points along the route to cheer me on and had been endlessly following the tracker, had arranged in advance for a beautiful pink bouquet to be sent to me and the flowers appeared as if by magic in the motorhome.

The original plan had been for Alan, Tim and I to spend the night in the motorhomes while Becky and Phil got lifts to their nearby homes. Instead we decided we would be much more comfortable in the Land's End Hotel. As we checked in, my legs seized up and Tim had to carry me to our room like I was a frail old woman. I had to be lifted in and out of the bath as I didn't have the strength to do it myself and I kept my eyes closed the whole time as I couldn't bear to look at my swollen, naked body. Once washed, I sank into the bed for the most welcome sleep of my life.

Even though I was exhausted, my body clock was still in JOGLE mode and I was wide awake at 4.30 a.m., thinking it was time to run again. It was a huge relief when I remembered it was over – I had done it. But I couldn't get back to sleep. Tim was fast asleep snoring loudly beside me so I reached for my laptop and began reading all the messages people had left me over the course of the challenge. I couldn't believe how many people had taken the time to contact me and donate money to Beat. There were messages from friends and family, acquaintances I hadn't been in touch with for years and dozens from people who I had never met who had been inspired by my story. Tears rolled down my cheeks as I read all their words of support, encouragement and congratulations. It was extraordinary how many people had been following my journey. I checked my Just Giving account and was overwhelmed by their generosity. I had raised £15,500 for the charity that was so close to my heart. That made all the pain I had been through worthwhile.

When Tim woke up, we headed for breakfast but it took a long time for me to get there. Anyone who has ever run a marathon will know how sore and stiff you can feel the next day – imagine what it is like after running 32 of them back to back. I could barely move as every muscle ached. I didn't actually feel that hungry but managed some bacon and eggs before we headed home. I was so tired on the route I barely had the energy to talk but I mustered a few words when a local radio station in Kent called to interview me. They congratulated me on my achievement, although I had to remind them the record wasn't official yet as all the evidence of the run had to be sent to Guinness World Records, with every mile accounted for, before it could be ratified. It would take weeks to pull together all the information required by Guinness, including signed witness statements of people who had seen me along the route, a detailed logbook of our journey, photos, press coverage and the GPS data from my tracker. Alan had written a supporting statement to add to the dossier and I was touched when I read what he had written, especially as I was not the first person he had helped achieve a JOGLE world record.

During the last three days of the challenge I have never witnessed such a determined and gutsy effort and Mimi's willingness to follow her crew's instructions and have faith in their calculations, without complaint nor query, was truly remarkable.

Six weeks after the evidence was sent in, I received a brown A4 envelope in the post that looked like an important document and I knew it had to be from Guinness World Records. I held it in my hands full of trepidation. This was it – the moment of truth. I almost couldn't open it. What if it said for some reason that I hadn't got the record? With a deep breath, I took the plunge and opened the envelope. I jumped up and down and squealed with delight as I pulled out a certificate topped with the Guinness World Record logo proclaiming:

The fastest confirmed journey from John o'Groats to Land's End on foot by a woman is 12 days, 15 hours, 46 minutes, 35 seconds by Marina Anderson (UK) from 16–28 July 2008.

Underneath was a stamp to say it was approved by Guinness World Records Ltd. The moment was overwhelming; I burst into tears (again!). It was official, I was a Guinness World Record holder. Tim and the rest of the crew were the first people I told the good news to, after all this record was theirs as much as mine and without their support I wouldn't have been able to achieve my dream. My mother and my children were also a massive part of my success. Even though they hadn't been part of the crew, they had been with me all the way in spirit. Their support and belief in me had been unconditional and I knew how proud they were of me.

. We had the certificate framed and hung on the kitchen wall. It was our victory. After keeping Tim separate from my running for so long and believing it was 'my thing', he had seamlessly become a member of my crew, saying and doing exactly the right thing at the right time. If he hadn't been there to urge me to keep going when I broke down in the last mile, I'll never know if I would have been able to finish. Such was the tired state of my brain at that time, I'd actually completely forgotten about the moment I wanted to quit – until Tim reminded me. He was keen to tell me it was 'just as well' he was there and I couldn't disagree. His involvement was a revelation and from then on, I would never shut him out of my race plans again. So as well as making me a world-record holder, JOGLE made my already strong marriage even stronger, proving without a doubt that Tim and I make a great team.

Receiving that certificate was amazing and there was an added thrill to come when I made it into the published version of the *Guinness Book of Records* in 2012 and 2013. Only nine per cent of the records set around the world make it into the annual publication so I was over the moon when I received an email from Guinness saying they were going to include the details of my JOGLE record. Ruaraidh had grown up enjoying reading the book, and now his mother was in it! It just goes to show what you can do with hard work, dedication and support.

I felt a huge sense of achievement and pride at gaining the record. It had been a goal I had been working towards for so long and the training and the challenge itself had taken a tremendous amount of time and energy. I definitely needed a break from running afterwards – both mentally and physically – but I wasn't planning to hang up my trainers for good. My desire to run and motivation to keep doing more challenges was still high. Before JOGLE, I had already signed up to run the Cape Odyssey, a five-day staged race held in the Western Cape of South Africa, running as a team with a friend. It was 12 weeks after JOGLE so I knew I wouldn't be fully recovered by then but I decided to just go there and enjoy the experience of running in a country that I loved. In the end, my friend was unable to make it so I was paired up with a mad Irishman living in Johannesburg called Ray Cranson. The whole race reminded me that running can just be for fun, it isn't always about chasing records and winning.

Before I started training for that, I took a few weeks off running – during which time I wouldn't have been capable of running even if I had wanted to. Once I was able to look at my trainers again with affection, I knew it was time to hit the trails again and I resumed some easy runs. As my body recovered and the swelling went down, it became evident how much weight I had lost during the JOGLE fortnight. When I made the rare decision to weigh myself, I was shocked to discover I had lost more than a stone. Despite eating what I thought was enough food, I had still struggled to take on enough calories. That was a lesson I would take forward to future challenges – I would have to eat more calorific, running-friendly foods. I knew it wasn't healthy to lose that much weight on a long-distance run as it meant my body hadn't just been burning fuel from food or fat stores to keep going. It had been forced to 'cannibalise' and burn muscle in its desperate attempt to convert energy to keep me moving.

As well as noticing my weight loss when I braved the scales, I noticed how thin I had become when I saw my reflection in the full-length mirror on our landing one day not long after JOGLE. I gasped when I saw my legs beneath my summer skirt. They were pin thin, completely stripped of all fat and muscle. I was captivated. These were the legs I had always dreamed of. Staring at this manifestation of what had been my goal for so long when I had an eating disorder, I realised how completely unrealistic and unhealthy my mindset for all those years had been. It had taken running 840 miles virtually non-stop for almost a fortnight to achieve what I once thought of as the 'perfect' legs. How crazy is that? No wonder I had never been able to achieve it before. And now looking at the legs I had always longed for, I realised I didn't actually want them after all. They may have been thin but they were frail. I couldn't run a marathon with these legs, they had no strength, no muscle – these legs were useless to me. Achieving a world record, along with all the other running goals I had met, meant so much more to me than having thin legs. Now I would much rather have toned, muscular legs, legs that could carry me over mountains, across deserts and the length of Great Britain in record time. I finally realised strong and healthy was a hundred times better than thin and frail. I didn't want to keep these 'perfect' skinny legs. I wanted to get back to running and make them sturdy and athletic again. Although I had physically beaten anorexia a long time ago, this was perhaps the moment I truly mentally conquered it as I realised how ridiculous my quest for the 'perfect' legs had been.

I know by beating anorexia I am one of the lucky ones, as it has a high mortality rate. Due to associated medical complications and suicide, 10 per cent of anorexia sufferers will die prematurely as a result of their illness. Approximately 1.6 million people in the UK suffer from an eating disorder and many of them will be suffering in silence. It not only affects them but the people who love them who can often only watch as their son, daughter, husband, wife, sibling or friend wastes away and they feel powerless to help.

Similar to being an alcoholic, often the person can't be helped until they acknowledge they have a problem. The only advice I can offer to people watching their loved one in this situation is don't try to force them to eat – this could only make them rebel. I would recommend seeking advice from a charity such as Beat, who I raised money for during JOGLE. They offer numerous support services from helplines to peer support groups. If you are someone who thinks they may have an eating disorder, then I also urge you to contact them, especially if you don't feel you can tell any of your friends and family. I know it is difficult but you must remember you are not alone and you can get better. I am proof this terrible illness can be overcome.

Completing JOGLE, gaining a world record and putting anorexia behind me highlighted just how far I had come. From that unhealthy mother with low self-confidence, who believed happiness was having thin legs and could barely run for a minute, I had become a formidable champion, an ultrarunner extraordinaire, capable of completing running feats I was told were impossible. Thanks to running, I now ooze happiness, confidence and self-belief. A desire for slimmer legs may have started my journey to become a runner but taking up the sport has changed so much more than my figure – it has changed my life.

CHAPTER SEVEN

SEEING DOUBLE AFTER JOGLE

After JOGLE my motivation and self-belief were high and I embarked on a series of new challenges – including a spate of 'doing the double' at some of the world's toughest ultra-races. In 2009, I ran Double Comrades in South Africa (112 miles); in 2011, I returned to Badwater to do the double there in order to try to break the current female record (292 miles); in 2013, I was the first person to complete the double at the Grand Union Canal Race (290 miles); and in 2015, I ran the Spartathlon in Greece twice (a total of 306 miles). Each of these challenges involved taking part in the race with the other competitors, having a very small break after the finish and then turning around to do the entire course again in reverse, just me and my support crew. Many people thought I was mad for doing this, as completing these races at all is enough of a challenge. But I felt if I was going to travel all that way to run, and spend a lot of money in the process, I needed an extra element to justify it. I also loved the idea of finding out what my body and mind were capable of and seeing if I could complete the most gruelling races in the world, not once, but twice. Each time I didn't know if doing the double was possible, but I reasoned I wouldn't know what I was capable of unless I tried, so I had to give it a go.

Each one of them was gruelling and difficult in its own way and the support of my crews was an intrinsic part of my success every time. At Comrades, it was as much of a logistic challenge as a physical one. The 56-mile race is run between the cities of Pietermaritzburg and Durban, each year alternating between runners racing 'up' from Durban to Pietermaritzburg or 'down' from Pietermaritzburg to Durban. The route incorporates five big hills that feel more like mountains but the inclines and declines are longer depending on the direction run. As I wouldn't have the support of the race organisers for one half of my challenge, I would need to arrange a crew and armed security guards to accompany me for safety, as well as informing the police of my intentions. The list was endless and I had to do it all from the other side of the world.

As the 2009 race course was a 'down' year, I decided to begin by doing the half of the double where I wouldn't join in the official race first, so I could get the 'uphill' route out of the way. I started my run the afternoon before the actual race from Durban and ran with my marvellous friend Neil Kapoor. With the help of my wonderful crew, I reached Pietermaritzburg in time to have a quick massage and something to eat before joining the official race start to go all the way back to Durban. I found doing the double this way round 'easier', as it meant I had other runners around me to chat to and the full support of the race organisers during the second part of the double when I was more fatigued.

Comrades is famous for its strict cut-off times along the course – five to be exact – and if you are one second late getting to one, that's it, you're out of the race, there is no leeway. This creates a huge spectacle of drama and heartbreak at the finish line as anyone who has managed to survive all the other time cut-offs must then finish within 12 hours in order to gain a medal. As the clock by the finish ticks closer to the 12-hour mark, an official stands holding a gun in the air with their back to the finishers. As soon as the second hand ticks over to 12 hours, the gun is fired, signalling the end of the race. It doesn't matter if you are a second away from the line – if you didn't cross it before the gun fired, you can't be an official finisher. My heart goes out to all those runners every year who work so hard to cover the 56 miles of hilly terrain, only to be denied a finishing medal because they just missed out on crossing the line in time. Thankfully, I didn't find out how this feels as I completed the 'up' run in 9 hours and 50 minutes, before turning back to finish the official race in 10 hours and 40 minutes, becoming the first woman to complete the Double Comrades, running a total of 112 miles.

Attempting Double Badwater had been on my radar since 2006 when I returned to the race to crew for Neil Kapoor. In 2011, the opportunity to do it myself was presented when I was one of the lucky people to be offered a place in the race. I knew how fortunate I was to be offered one of the coveted places – and remembered how hard I had worked to earn one in 2005, so I felt I couldn't turn it down. After studying Ben Jones's comprehensive list of every Badwater finisher, including people who have achieved double, triple and even quadruple crossings, I found the female record for the double was within my capabilities so I decided to go for it. The double would involve running the challenging 135-mile race followed by a 22-mile run/hike up and down Mount Whitney – the highest mountain in the contiguous USA – before running all the way back to the start at Badwater Basin, a grand total of 292 miles. I would have to do it in less than 129 hours – just over five and a half days – to break the record.

Doing the double at Badwater wasn't a decision I made lightly, and I'm sure many people thought, once again, that I was crazy. I wouldn't have even considered it if I hadn't run the race before but I knew the route and the conditions so I had a good idea what to expect. I knew one of the biggest hurdles would be staying hydrated so I spent weeks acclimatising in a sauna again as part of my preparation.

On race day, thanks to the support of my crew – Becky again, Katherine Hay-Heddle, Matt Nelson, Brad Lombardi and Will Glover – who constantly sprayed me with water during the hottest parts of the race, I crossed the finish line in a respectable time of 34 hours and 25 minutes, finishing 24th overall and 4th female. It had been a tricky one to pace as I wanted to be competitive while still leaving myself enough in the tank for the return journey. Before turning back, I had to scale Mount Whitney. It was this part of the double that really excited me as I had never climbed that high before. It was also the most critical part of the journey, as if the weather was too bad, the road would be closed preventing me from going for the record. Just days before, it had been shut due to heavy snow but by the time we were due to climb, it was safe to be reopened to hikers. The ascent involves making lots of switchback turns as it is so steep before a final scramble to the summit. Reaching the peak was a life-affirming moment. I felt on top of the world looking down on the stunning views below. Standing there above the clouds at 14,500 feet, a sense of tranquillity and calm embraced me. Despite my tiredness, I felt invincible and I was ready to take on the second stage of the race.

The run back felt completely different to the race experience as there were no other runners or their crews around to distract me. It was just me, my crew and the never-ending open road. My pace started to slow due to a nagging blister, but as I reached each checkpoint, my crew told me I was still on target to beat the previous record, which incentivised me to keep going. Runners on their way home passed me in their cars and would toot their horns as they passed or wind down their windows to shout words of encouragement. A few even stopped to get out of their cars to have a chat and see how I was doing, it was all very supporting and encouraging. Each toot or shout out of a window lifted my spirits and spurred me on. The greatest moment of the return journey was just before Stove Pipe Wells where I was due to have a short rest. It made my day when Marshall Ulrich himself drove past, stopped in the middle of the road and got out of his car to speak to me. Marshall is a Badwater legend, a former race victor. He has finished it countless times, including doing the quadruple. His long list of achievements also includes ascending Mount Everest and doing a record-breaking 3,000-mile run across America from San Francisco to New York City. He's one of my running heroes so I was completely star-struck when he pulled over to stop and speak to me. He said I was much further along the route than he expected, you can imagine how thrilled I was to hear this. To have so far exceeded his expectations was unbelievable.

The miles rolled by and eventually the finish was in sight, I mustered all the last energy I had to pick up the pace and cross the line. There were no cheering crowds and no finishing tape to break but while the end may have lacked atmosphere, I was ecstatic when I checked the time. I had finished in 108 hours, 10 minutes and 24 seconds (around four and a half days), beating the previous female record by over 21 hours! I was also the first British female to complete the double. I had to keep pinching myself, I just couldn't believe I had done it. My crew wrapped a union flag around my shoulders and I held it aloft as I posed for pictures like an Olympian doing their lap of honour after winning a gold medal.

While I managed to dig deep to do the double at Comrades and Badwater on my first attempts, the double Spartathlon was much harder to achieve and I failed in my first bid in 2013. The Spartathlon is one of the most iconic races in the ultrarunning world. It's 153 miles non-stop from Athens to Sparta, imitating a route that was said to have been taken by Pheidippides in ancient Greece. He was a messenger sent to deliver news of a victory against the Persians at the battle of Marathon, and died from exhaustion after completing the epic journey on foot. The story became the inspiration for the marathon, even though Pheidippides ran further than 26.2 miles.

In 1982, John Foden, a British RAF wing commander who was a fan of ancient Greek history, wondered if it really was possible for a man to run 153 miles within 36 hours on the same terrain Pheidippides covered. He decided to put the legend to the test and the Spartathlon was born.

Modern-day competitors following in Pheidippides' footsteps have to run on rough tracks, through olive groves and up and down steep hillsides before tackling the 4,000-ft ascent and descent of Mount Parthenion to finish in Sparta, where it is tradition to finish by running up the steps and kissing the foot of the statue of King Leonidas. To make it even tougher there are 74 checkpoints along the route, each with its own cut-off time, so competitors are constantly chasing the clock. Less than half the field of runners usually make it to the finish line.

I completed the race in 2011, coming third female, and this gave me the confidence to go back in 2013 to try to become the first woman to achieve the double crossing. I planned to run the race, then turn round and run all the way back to Athens. Unfortunately due to a variety of things, including not consuming enough food on the run, as I approached the last stage of the race, I started getting slower and slower. With ten miles to go to the finish of the official race, my body bent over backwards and I turned into a rag doll. Medics rushed to help me and I could only manage to stay upright with their support. I was timed out of the race and had to be driven to the finish line. I was devastated. On that occasion, I hadn't managed to finish the Spartathlon once, let alone twice. Although this attempt at the double was an epic failure, I didn't stay down about it for long. I believe you can always turn a negative into a positive if you're willing to learn from your mistakes. My crew and I returned in 2015 and this time I did become the first female to complete the Double Spartathlon. It was one of my proudest achievements as I hadn't given up when at first I hadn't succeeded. I had come back stronger and proved to myself I could do it.

While these double challenges whet my competitive appetite and truly tested my physical and mental capabilities, I was also keen to go for more world records. JOGLE hadn't just been about the desire to succeed; I had also enjoyed the planning aspect, working out how to manage my body, when to eat and to sleep, decisions that were pivotal to success or failure.

In 2010, I decided to go for another world record, this time on a treadmill. I wanted to try to get the record for the longest distance covered by a female running on a treadmill for seven days. The record at the time stood at 395 miles – meaning I would have to run more than two marathons a day in order to break it, allowing myself just two hours' sleep each day. Although I had my sights set on breaking the female record, I also knew I had a chance of beating the male record, which was then 517 miles. I knew I was capable of this mileage; the biggest issue in this world-record attempt would be beating the boredom.

After discovering a love of running outdoors, using a treadmill was something I had always tried to avoid. I'll only use one if the weather outside is very icy, and the maximum I can bear is an hour. Treadmill, or dreadmill running as I prefer to call it, always seems to go incredibly slowly, while an hour running outside passes by in a flash, as I'm busy enjoying my surroundings. I knew running on the treadmill for a week would be a huge challenge for me.

For a treadmill world-record attempt, Guinness insists that the challenge takes place in a public area. I asked the Ashford Designer Outlet, a shopping centre near my home in Kent, whether they would accommodate me for a week and thankfully they agreed. This venue is always teeming with shoppers who would be able to give me lots of support and a fantastic distraction from the relentless monotonous miles running on the treadmill. Even when the outlet was closed to shoppers I would be entertained by the workmen swinging from ropes as they repaired the tent-like roof, or I'd chat to the security guards as they did their rounds. I also had company from the amazing people supporting me; some were there for the duration and others popped in once or twice a day to bring me treats to eat, which was always a highlight and very much appreciated.

I had a second treadmill set up alongside mine for two reasons. Firstly, if my machine broke down I could quickly switch to the other one, and secondly it enabled friends to run alongside me to keep me sane and share some of my pain. It's this kind of support that makes a real difference when going through a bad patch.

While this record attempt didn't involve difficult terrain, adverse weather conditions or navigating a route like some of my previous races, it was still one of the hardest things

I have ever done. At the end of the first day I developed a stress fracture in my foot – basically I had broken my toe. A podiatrist assessed my foot and recommended I stop running and pull out of the record attempt, but this wasn't an option for me. The attempt was on and I was running for Help for Heroes. With so much money at stake for a good cause, I had no intention of dropping out. My foot was taped up and I was given new trainers half a size bigger in order to try to make running feel easier as my foot had become so swollen.

While I wasn't going to quit because of the stress fracture, it meant I had no choice but to re-evaluate my running goal. The pain in my foot impacted on my pace, and at times I was reduced to a shuffle. I wasn't going fast enough to break the male record but if I pushed hard enough, I could still take the female one. The pain each time my broken foot landed altered my running gait so I wasn't able to flow as naturally as I usually ran. This caused blisters to develop and caused my foot to become even more inflamed, inflating by a further two shoe sizes.

But one day turned into the next and as I kept running, the record was within my grasp, I tried to block the pain out and carry on. The local BBC news heard about this mad woman running for seven days on a treadmill and came along to film me. When they arrived I was about to take a short break for a much-needed massage so the camera crew were treated to a look at my battered feet. I'm sure viewers didn't appreciate seeing a close up of my blisters as they ate their dinner watching the six o'clock news!

By the last day, I was on target to beat the female record, I just had to keep going until midday. As the minutes ticked down, I drew a crowd who spurred me on to pick up the pace for the final two minutes. They gave me a ten-second countdown and cheered and applauded when the clock struck 12 and I was able to stop. It was such an emotional moment. As usual I couldn't hold back the tears of joy and relief as people congratulated me, including the mayor of Ashford who handed me a bouquet of flowers – pink, of course! I had run 403.81 miles achieving a new female world record. I punched the air in triumph and stepped off the treadmill – vowing never to step on one ever again!

This record has since been broken but I don't mind at all. As far as I am concerned, records are there to be smashed. I believe whoever holds a record is merely looking after it until passing it on to the next worthy person. I am still 'looking after' the JOGLE world record, as that is yet to be beaten. I would have the utmost respect for anyone who does it as I know just how much training and effort is involved.

I also still have another world record to my name – the fastest crossing of Ireland on foot by a female. Having run the length of the UK, it seemed only sensible to try to run the length of Ireland as well. The attempt was decided when

I was sitting with Becky and Katherine enjoying a coffee in Furnace Creek the day after they had helped me complete the Double Badwater.

'So, what's your next venture going to be?' Katherine asked me, knowing full well I would already have something in mind, despite my body still aching from just finishing another colossal challenge.

'Coast to coast across Ireland?' I suggested.

Without batting an eyelid, they both immediately signed up as crew. A year later, after months of planning and training, we were ready to start the world-record attempt, starting at Malin Head in County Donegal and finishing at Mizen Head in County Cork, a total distance of 345 miles. Tim joined Becky and Katherine on the crew. They were all so experienced at aiding my running by then, they seamlessly slotted into their roles, making everything run like clockwork when we set off on 22 September 2012.

Unlike JOGLE, there were no car collisions, no police hold-ups and no mental meltdowns from me. It was one of those rare races when everything went to plan and the angels were definitely smiling down on me. I felt great and I finished feeling as though I had given my all. Of course, running 345 miles against the clock was still very hard work, but when it got tough, I kept focusing on what it would mean to finish and achieve another record.

The beautiful scenery in Ireland and the friendly people who made me feel very welcome also helped. Groups of runners would appear on the roadside every day to run with me for a couple of hours. My crew motivated me by making signs out of silver duct tape telling me how far I had to go, which they would stick to the back of the motorhome. *200 miles to go, 100 miles to go, 50 miles to go*; every time I saw the smaller number, it gave me such a boost.

The final section was the most painful and during the agonising last two miles the finish line never seemed to get any closer. Katherine, who was cycling with me at the time, and I began to wonder if we had gone the wrong way. Finally we made it to Mizen Head and another world-record dream came true as I finished in 3 days, 15 hours, 36 minutes and 23 seconds. I hadn't just achieved the record, but smashed it by just over 10 hours.

Along with the doubles and world records, over the past ten years I've also taken part in more desert ultras, the Ice Ultra, mountain races and, in 2012, I even competed in the Jungle Ultra, a 143-mile, five-day self-sufficiency race through the Peruvian jungle. I can't tell you how many bugs there are in the jungle, many of them designed to eat humans! There were also endless river crossings to deal with, unbearable humidity and torrential rain. It well and truly took me out of my comfort zone but it was a real privilege to run in a part of the world few people venture into, and I was delighted to finish first female.

Another standout event was the Libyan Challenge, which I was invited to take part in in 2006. It's not exactly a holiday destination, so I couldn't turn down the opportunity to go there. The race involves running through the Sahara again, this time doing 120 miles non-stop through the Tadrart Acacus region. This area is a World Heritage Site famous for two things – thousands of prehistoric cave paintings dating back to 12,000 BC, and its jagged lunar landscape with towering granite mountains stretching 5,000 ft into the sky. Usually you can only see the landmarks with a guide but we were to run through this magnificent place using our own GPS watches for guidance.

It was the first time I had used a GPS to help me navigate a run, and I was a little sceptical at first and feared the technology would let me down, but it served me well and I never got lost – which was a massive relief when running through the desert in the pitch black of night. The route involved rock climbing, with some dangerous descents, and crossing huge expanses of sand, with no respite from the heat of the sun, often accompanied by masses of flies that must be fans of the smell of sweat!

The various rock formations I passed along the way were incredible. Some resembled cathedrals, others ships, and my favourite was one called the Elephant Foot which looked exactly as if an elephant had stomped its foot into the sand and left it there, separated from its body from the sole to the knee. I felt so lucky to be able to run through such a place, joining forces with three other women from different countries who were taking part to finish as joint first ladies.

I returned to Africa in 2014 for what would be my greatest challenge there yet. After two years of planning I ran 1,223 miles over 32 days along the Freedom Trail in South Africa with my friend Samantha Gash. The route was set up as a mountain bike race and I believe we were only the third people to have run the course that begins in Pietermaritzburg and finishes in Paarl, just outside Cape Town.

The trail, made up of dirt roads and cattle tracks, wasn't clearly marked so it was difficult to navigate and at times the path disappeared altogether so we frequently got lost. Along the route we traversed the high mountains of Lesotho, the wide open spaces of the Karoo and six mountain ranges. We also ran through endless beautiful valleys, national parks and nature reserves. Running through the private game reserves always kept us on our toes as we never knew when we would see a wild animal. Thankfully the rhinos we passed were secured behind a high wire fence but the warthogs and antelopes ran free, often crossing our path. We were told a leopard lived in the final valley we ran through but sadly we never saw him. It was an amazing experience and a privilege to run through such a magnificent country.

I'm often asked why I run and it is partly for opportunities like these, to be able to go out and have an adventure exploring otherwise forgotten places and remote landscapes, experiencing different cultures and meeting inspirational people along the way. On a day-to-day basis, I run simply because I love it. It makes me feel alive, giving me the freedom and space to have my own thoughts. I also run because I can, and I know how lucky I am to be able to. Running has made me happy and healthy and helped me put anorexia firmly in its place.

EPILOGUE

I am 55 years old now and a grandmother of three. Despite everything I have achieved so far, I'm still not ready to stop pushing myself. In fact, I am currently planning my biggest challenge to date – running across America, which has been a dream of mine for years. In September 2017, I intend to start my run on the steps of the City Hall in Los Angeles and run across 12 states to finish on the steps of New York City Hall, approximately 2,850 miles later. It will be the furthest I have ever run and, of course, there will be no time for sightseeing, as I hope to set a new female world record. The current one was set by a South African woman called Mavis Hutchison, who completed her crossing in 69 days and 2 hours back in 1979, which just goes to show how tough this record is to break. I've been planning the record attempt for more than two years – there's a full-size map of the USA hanging on my kitchen wall with my route plotted out and it's a very long way! My 'A goal' is to run across this massive country in under 53 days, leaving enough of a cushion to still break the record if the unexpected happens – which of course it's bound to, given the distance I'm planning to run. A crew of five will be there to support me, one of whom I am hoping will be a physiotherapist. With a bit of luck, Tim will be able to join me for a few weeks towards the end if things aren't too busy for him at work. Running the length of Great Britain has been the toughest thing I have ever done and running across America will be even harder, so it's not something I'm taking on lightly. Am I mad to try it? Perhaps, especially as at the time of writing this book, I have been recovering from a knee operation to repair torn cartilage in the joint. It took four months of rest and rehab before I could finally get back into training. Although this book has largely been about my successes, I've had my fair share of failures too, from the aborted first JOGLE world-record attempt to dropping out of races due to injury. I know a lot could go wrong in my bid to become the fastest female to run across America. JOGLE taught me that plans always need to be adaptable in order to succeed. The road ahead is long and I know it won't be easy but I have to give it a go. Some will say it's impossible, but of course I don't believe that. As one of my favourite quotes by Arthur C. Clarke states: 'The only limitations you have in life are the ones you put on yourself.'

MIMI'S ULTRARUNNING ACHIEVEMENTS SO FAR...

2001

Thames Meander, 54-mile race from Reading to London.
Marathon des Sables, 155-mile race in the Sahara desert.

2002

Trailwalker UK, 62-mile race over the South Downs from Queen Elizabeth Country Park, Hampshire to Brighton race course, fastest mixed team.

2003

Marathon of Britain, 175-mile, seven-day staged race from Warwickshire to Nottingham, 3rd fastest female.

2004

Himalayan 100, 100-mile, five-day staged, 3rd fastest female.

Rome Marathon, 26.2 miles. PB: 3 hours 34 minutes.

Grand Union Canal Race, 145-mile non-stop from Birmingham to London, 15th overall out of 23 finishers (54 runners started the race), 2nd fastest female, finishing time: 39 hours 39 minutes.

2005

Badwater Ultramarathon, 135 miles, starting in Death Valley and finishing in the Mount Witney Portals, USA, 23rd overall, 6th fastest female, 1st Brit, 41 hours 5 minutes 35 seconds.

Paris to London, 330 miles, including marathons in both cities.

2006

Kalahari Augrabies Extreme Marathon, 155-mile, self-sufficiency desert race over seven days, 6th overall, 1st female, finishing time: 31 hours 46 minutes.

Pennine 100 Pursuit, 62 miles, 4th overall out of eight finishers (29 competitors started the event), 1st female, 1st female vet (aged 40 and over).

Libyan Challenge Master Trek, 120-mile non-stop self-sufficiency desert race over four days, 3rd overall, 1st female.

Tring 2 Town, 40 miles from London's Little Venice to Tring, 2nd female, 1st female vet.

2007

CHAMPION AND COURSE RECORD: *6633 Arctic Ultra*, a 352-mile self-sufficiency race in the Arctic over eight days. I won in 143 hours 23 minutes – just under six days, coming in 24 hours ahead of the next person. I am the only female to have finished so far and still hold the course record.

Seni Extreme, 200-mile non-stop race from Dudley just north of Birmingham to the ExCel in London. I won in 67 hours 13 minutes.

2008

FEMALE WORLD RECORD JOGLE, beginning in John O'Groats all the way to Land's End, 840 miles in total over 12 days, finishing time: 12 days, 15 hours 46 minutes.

Cape Odyssey, five-day staged race held in the Western Cape of South Africa run in teams of pairs. My team finished 53rd out of 164.

Atacama Crossing, 150-mile self-sufficiency staged race in the Atacama Desert, Chile, 20th overall, 1st female.

Tring 2 Town 'Double', 80 miles, 2nd female, 1st female vet.

Thames Path Challenge, 50-mile race from Reading to Shepperton, with navigation as the Thames was flooded so we had to find our own routes, 2nd female, finishing time: 7 hours 48 minutes.

2009

FIRST FEMALE TO COMPLETE DOUBLE COMRADES, 56 miles from Durban to Pietermaritzburg in 9 hours 50 minutes, followed by joining in the official race to run back again in 10 hours 40 minutes, covering a total of 112 miles.

The Druid's Challenge, 82-mile, three-day event along the Ridgeway, from Wiltshire to Buckinghamshire, 25th overall.

Kalahari Augrabies Extreme Marathon, finished in 27 hours 5 minutes, 10th overall, 1st female.

Al Andalus Ultimate Trail, Spain, 62-mile staged race over five days, 1st female, 8th overall.

Tring 2 Town Double, 80 miles, 8th overall, 1st female.

2010

FEMALE TREADMILL WORLD RECORD, furthest distance covered on a treadmill in seven days by a female, a total of 403.81 miles (this record has since been broken).

FEMALE COURSE RECORD GRAND UNION CANAL RACE, 145 miles non-stop from Birmingham to London. I came in 3rd overall, setting a new record for women in 28 hours and 12 minutes.

Namibian Desert Challenge, 136-mile, five-day self-sufficiency staged race, won overall, finishing time: 25 hours 23 minutes.

2011

FEMALE COURSE RECORD AND FIRST BRITISH FEMALE TO COMPLETE DOUBLE BADWATER, ran the Badwater Ultramarathon (135 miles), then climbed to the top of Mount Whitney (14,505 ft above sea level, 11 miles), then all the way back to the start of the original race at Badwater, a total distance of 292 miles. I finished in 108 hours and 10 minutes beating the previous female record by more than 21 hours and becoming the first British female to complete the double.

Spartathlon, 153-mile non-stop race from Athens to Sparta in under 36 hours with cut-offs at every checkpoint. I finished 37th out of 285 starters (145 finishers), 3rd female and 1st Brit, with a finishing time of 32 hours 33 minutes.

Glenmore 24 Trail Race, as many laps of the 4-mile course as you can in 24 hours. I ran 112 miles, coming in 3rd overall and 1st female.

101 Ronda, 63-mile trail race in Spain to be completed in 24 hours, 3rd female, 2nd female vet, finishing time: 11 hours 31 minutes.

Glasgow to Edinburgh Ultramarathon, 56 miles along the canals, finished 11th overall and 1st female.

2012

WORLD RECORD, THE FASTEST CROSSING ON FOOT OF IRELAND, started in Malin Head and finished at Mizen Head, a total of 345 miles in three days, finishing time: 3 days, 15 hours 36 minutes 55 seconds.

Jungle Ultra Marathon, 146-mile, six-day staged race in the jungle of Peru, 4th overall, 1st female.

Viking Way Ultra, 148-mile non-stop race starting at the Humber Bridge, Yorkshire, and finishing in Oakham, Rutland, 3rd overall, the only female to ever complete the course, finishing time: 33 hours 52 minutes.

Thames Path 100, 100-mile non-stop race starting at Richmond, London, and finishing in Oxford along the Thames Path, 7th overall, 1st female, finishing time: 18 hours 50 minutes.

2013

FIRST PERSON TO COMPLETE DOUBLE GRAND UNION CANAL RACE, a total of 290 miles running from Birmingham to London and back again, finishing time: 36 hours 49 minutes.

Mountain Ultra, 146-mile, five-day staged race in Colorado, USA, 2nd female.

2014

1,968 KM ON THE FREEDOM TRAIL, 1,223 miles run over 32 days in South Africa from Pietermaritzburg to Paarl, just outside Cape Town.

Cyprus Ultra, 135 miles non-stop. I was the only finisher, setting a new course record of 41 hours 34 minutes.

2015

Thames Path 100, 2nd female.

Grand Union Canal Race, 145 miles non-stop, 1st female.

Run the Rann, invited to test run the course for this inaugural 100-mile non-stop event in a remote area of India, run across salt flats, cliffs and through tonnes of thorny bushes.

FIRST FEMALE TO COMPLETE THE DOUBLE SPARTATHLON. I took part in the 153-mile non-stop race from Athens to Sparta with cut-offs at every checkpoint, finishing in 35 hours and 7 minutes. After a few hours' rest, I turned back to complete the course in reverse, running a total of 306 miles.

2016
Ice Ultra Marathon, 143-mile, self-sufficiency race through Arctic Sweden, 4th overall, 1st female.

2017
WORLD RECORD ATTEMPT: COAST TO COAST ACROSS THE USA. Starting in LA in September, I intend to run 2,850 miles to finish in New York, 53 days later (the current official record is 69 days).

FURTHER READING

For help and support regarding eating disorders, contact the charity Beat. Visit their website at **b-eat.co.uk**

For information on ultrarunning and global races, some useful websites include **ultramarathonrunning.com** and **runultra.co.uk**

The Trail Running Association website can be found at **tra-uk.org** and visit **centurionrunning.com** for trail ultramarathon events.

Visit **www.xnrg.co.uk** for information on fantastic multi-day events around the UK and the Isle of Wight.

For more information on some of the races featured in the book:

Marathon Des Sables: **marathondessables.com**
Badwater Ultramarathon: **badwater.com**
6633 Arctic Ultra: **6633ultra.com**
Grand Union Canal Race: **gucr.co.uk**
Kalahari Augrabies Extreme Marathon: **kaem.co.za**
Spartathlon: **spartathlon.gr/en**
Comrades Marathon: **comrades.com**
Himalayan 100: **himalayan.com**

For more information on Guinness World Records and how to attempt to break one visit **guinnessworldrecords.com**

Follow me on Twitter **@marvellousmimi** and via my website **marvellousmimi.com** for race updates.

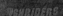

ADVENTUREMAN
Anyone Can Be a Superhero

Jamie McDonald

£9.99

Paperback

ISBN: 978-1-84953-969-2

When Jamie decides to repay the hospitals that saved his life as a child, he embarks on the biggest challenge of his life: running the equivalent of 200 marathons back-to-back, solo and unsupported, in −40 degree weather, surviving all kinds of injuries and traumas on the road and wearing through 13 pairs of trainers. And he does it all dressed as the superhero, the Flash.

Though his journey was both mentally and physically exhausting, it was the astounding acts of kindness and hospitality he encountered along the way that kept him going. Whether they gave him a bed for the night, food for the journey, a donation to his charity or companionship and encouragement during the long days of running, Jamie soon came to realise that every person who helped him towards his goal was a superhero too.

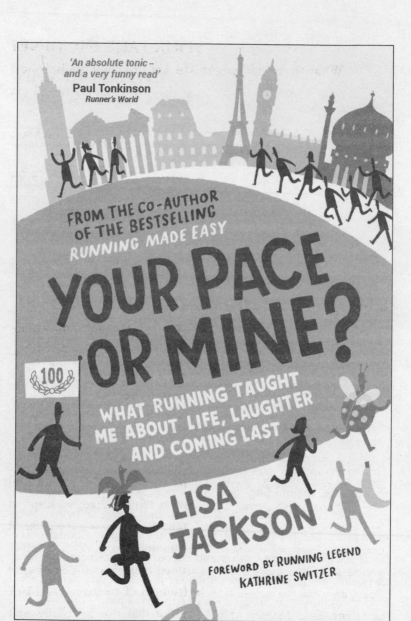

'An absolute tonic –
and a very funny read'
Paul Tonkinson
Runner's World

FROM THE CO-AUTHOR
OF THE BESTSELLING
RUNNING MADE EASY

YOUR PACE OR MINE?

100

WHAT RUNNING TAUGHT
ME ABOUT LIFE, LAUGHTER
AND COMING LAST

LISA JACKSON

FOREWORD BY RUNNING LEGEND
KATHRINE SWITZER

YOUR PACE OR MINE?
What Running Taught Me About Life, Laughter and Coming Last

Lisa Jackson

£9.99

Paperback

ISBN: 978-1-84953-827-5

Lisa Jackson is a surprising cheerleader for the joys of running. Formerly a committed fitness-phobe, she became a marathon runner at 31, and ran her first 56-mile ultramarathon aged 41. And unlike many runners, Lisa's not afraid to finish last – in fact, she's done so in 20 of the 90-plus marathons she's completed so far.

But this isn't just Lisa's story, it's also that of the extraordinary people she's met along the way – tutu-clad fun-runners, octogenarians, 250-mile ultrarunners – whose tales of loss and laughter are sure to inspire you just as much as they've inspired her. This book is for anyone who longs to experience the sense of connection and achievement that running has to offer, whether you're a nervous novice or a seasoned marathoner dreaming of doing an ultra. An account of the triumph of tenacity over a lack of talent, *Your Pace or Mine?* is proof that running really isn't about the time you do, but the time you have!

Have you enjoyed this book?
If so, why not write a review on your favourite website?

If you're interested in finding out more about our
books, find us on Facebook at **Summersdale Publishers**
and follow us on Twitter **@Summersdale.**

Thanks very much for buying this Summersdale book.

www.summersdale.com